MAYO CLINIC
— ON —
HEALTHY AGING

An Easy and Comprehensive Guide to
Keeping Your Body Young,
Your Mind Sharp and Your Spirit Fulfilled

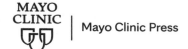 Mayo Clinic Press

MAYO CLINIC PRESS

Medical Editors Nathan K. LeBrasseur, Ph.D.,
Christina Chen, M.D.
Publisher Daniel J. Harke
Editor in Chief Nina E. Wiener
Senior Editor Karen R. Wallevand
Art Director Stewart J. Koski
Production Designer Darren L. Wendt
Illustration and Photography Mayo Clinic Media
Support Services, Mayo Clinic Medical Illustration
and Animation
Editorial Research Librarian Anthony J. Cook
Contributors Sophie J. Bakri, M.D.; Jamie M. Bogle,
Au.D., Ph.D.; William A. Brown, J.D.; Eduardo N. Chini,
M.D., Ph.D.; Edward T. Creagan, M.D.; Jorg Goronzy,
M.D., Ph.D.; Ryan T. Hurt, M.D., Ph.D.; Dona E. Locke,
Ph.D.; Alexander Meves, M.D., M.B.A.; Jordan D. Miller,
Ph.D.; Candace M. Nelson; Eric J. Olson, M.D.; Robert
J. Pignolo, M.D., Ph.D.; Sandhya Pruthi, M.D.; Daniel E.
Sanchez Pellecer, M.D.; Taryn L. Smith, M.D.; Ericka E.
Tung, M.D., M.P.H.; Stephanie K. Vaughan; Laura M.
Waxman

Additional contributions from Kirkus Reviews, Rachel
Lehmann-Haupt, Orvos Communications and Rath
Indexing

Image Credits All photographs and illustrations are
copyright of Mayo Foundation for Medical Education
and Research (MFMER) except for the following:
Cover/Credit: Sarayut Thaneerat/Moment via Getty
Images, Kampee Patisena/Moment via Getty Images;
Page 199/Credit: iStock.com/PeopleImages/iStock/
Getty Images Plus via Getty Images; Page 251/Credit:
Alina Kulbasnaia / iStock / Getty Images Plus via Getty
Images/keira01 / iStock / Getty Images Plus via Getty
Images/a_namenko / iStock / Getty Images Plus via
Getty Images/Aamulya / iStock / Getty Images Plus via
Getty Images/Mas Bro / 500px via Getty Images/
AnaBGD / iStock / Getty Images Plus via Getty Images

Published by Mayo Clinic Press

© 2024 Mayo Foundation for Medical Education and
Research (MFMER)

The information in this book is true and complete to
the best of our knowledge. This book is intended as an
informative guide for those wishing to learn more
about health issues. It is not intended to replace,
countermand or conflict with advice given to you by
your own physician. The ultimate decision concerning
your care should be made between you and your
doctor. Information in this book is offered with no
guarantees. The author and publisher disclaim all
liability in connection with the use of this book.

For bulk sales to employers, member groups and
health-related companies, contact Mayo Clinic,
200 First St. SW, Rochester, MN 55905, or send an
email to SpecialSalesMayoBooks@mayo.edu.

To stay informed about Mayo Clinic Press,
please subscribe to our free e-newsletter at
MCPress.MayoClinic.org or follow us on social media.

ISBN: 979-8-88770-023-6 (hardcover)
Library of Congress Control Number: 2023939869

Printed in the United States

Table of Contents

4   *Preface*

6   **Chapter 1:** Age*less* — longevity and how we age

18   **Part 1: Common age-related changes and what you can do**
19   **Chapter 2:** Your brain
44   **Chapter 3:** Your senses
60   **Chapter 4:** Your heart and lungs
84   **Chapter 5:** Your bones, muscles and joints
101   **Chapter 6:** Your digestive health
117   **Chapter 7:** Your urinary health
127   **Chapter 8:** Your immune health
135   **Chapter 9:** Weight, sleep, skin and sexual health
161   **Chapter 10:** Cancer
178   **Chapter 11:** Frailty and recovery from injury

186   **Part 2: Living better and living longer**
187   **Chapter 12:** How are you doing, and what's your plan?
196   **Chapter 13:** The power of relationships, connections and purpose
215   **Chapter 14:** Improving your physical health with exercise
249   **Chapter 15:** Eating well to live well
261   **Chapter 16:** Holistic health to nurture your mind, body and spirit
272   **Chapter 17:** Vaccinations and screening tests
296   **Chapter 18:** Planning ahead for what comes next
312   **Chapter 19:** Inspirational stories

319   *Additional resources*
323   *Index*

Preface

From Alzheimer's disease to osteoarthritis, having another birthday increases your risk of becoming a statistic. That's because the greatest risk factor for most chronic diseases is aging.

Your later years — those "golden years" — can be some of the best of your life. Unfortunately, while people today are generally living longer than in decades past, they aren't always living better. For many, the last decades of their lives are often racked with diseases and disabilities that diminish their quality of life.

Researchers at Mayo Clinic's Kogod Center on Aging are probing ways to help slow the clock on chronic conditions that set in as we get older. The aim of this research isn't to increase longevity — although living longer is certainly a possible outcome. Rather, the goal is to increase health span, the length of time that people remain relatively free of disease and disability, so that they can enjoy higher-quality lives.

Recent research suggests that aging may be a modifiable risk factor — in other words, a process that can be controlled. At Mayo Clinic, scientists are interested in learning more about the processes that lead to molecular and cellular damage associated with disease and illness as we mature.

In this book, we discuss what we currently know about the aging process and what you can expect to experience as you get older. More importantly, we outline ways that you can remain healthy as you age, so that your later years can be some of your best years.

Nathan LeBrasseur, Ph.D.
Christina Chen, M.D.

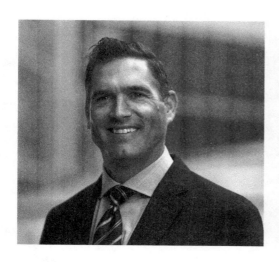

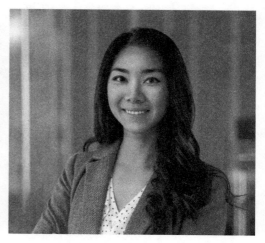

Nathan K. LeBrasseur, Ph.D., is the director of the Robert and Arlene Kogod Center on Aging, the co-director of the Paul F. Glenn Center for Biology of Aging Research, and the scientific director of the Office of Translation to Practice at Mayo Clinic. A professor of physical medicine and rehabilitation and associate professor of physiology in the Mayo Clinic College of Medicine and Science, he also serves as the current chair of the NIH Cellular Mechanisms in Aging and Development Study Section. Dr. LeBrasseur is a recipient of the Glenn Award for Research in Biological Mechanisms of Aging, the Nathan W. Shock Award Lecture from the National Institute on Aging, and the Vincent Cristofalo Rising Star Award in Aging Research from the American Federation for Aging Research. He is a Fellow of the Gerontological Society of America.

Christina Chen, M.D., is a geriatrician in the division of Community Internal Medicine, Geriatrics and Palliative Care at Mayo Clinic in Rochester, Minn., with a dual appointment in Integrative Medicine and Health, where she trained in acupuncture. Dr. Chen is involved in a variety of educational endeavors, including course director for geriatrics curriculum (Senior Sages Program) at the Mayo Clinic Alix School of Medicine, didactic core curriculum leader for the Geriatrics Medicine Fellowship, and course director for the Care of the Older Adult, a continuing medical education conference. Her research focus is on transforming dementia care through integrative therapies and environmental redesign and she has led several clinical trials. Dr. Chen is the host of the Mayo Clinic podcast, "Aging Forward."

Ageless — longevity and how we age

At age 101, one of Rachel's favorite mottos is "Don't let anybody get you down, never be pessimistic and work for the best."

It's a lifelong attitude that was born out of early tragedy. At age 15, Rachel was rescued from Nazi Germany, where her family perished. She was brought to what is now Israel, where she met the man who became her husband of more than 64 years. Eventually, the couple made their way to the United States to further their educations. Rachel studied art and went on to make paintings, prints and sculptures. At the same time, she built a rewarding career teaching Hebrew to children and selling houses as a real estate agent.

Visiting with Rachel is a fascinating lesson in perseverance, resilience and healthy living. Her enormous strength through adversity and her full engagement with life are part of what has kept her young at heart. Throughout her life, she's also made her health a priority.

Rachel believes a factor integral to her long life is her diet. She makes a point to eat plenty of vegetables and fruits. "I try to stay away from red meat," she says. To ensure she gets enough protein, Rachel includes chicken, fish, eggs and yogurt in her meals. She especially enjoys bean chili and chicken soup, and her favorite weekend meal is bagels and smoked salmon. She also savors a sweet treat now and then — especially chocolate.

Rachel recalls that when her husband was alive, the two of them would sometimes enjoy half a glass of wine together. But she says that nowadays, she doesn't drink any alcohol. "I want to keep my mind clear," she remarks.

Another constant in Rachel's long life has been physical activity. "I was four years old when I learned to swim, and I've been swimming ever since." For years, Rachel swam six days a week at her local YMCA. She and her husband were also avid downhill skiers. Their annual visits to ski resorts were the highlight of their winters. More recently, Rachel started working with a personal trainer, who has guided her in weekly strengthening exercises, including exercises for legs, arms and hands.

In addition to her physical health, Rachel strives to keep her mind sharp. A lifelong reader, she spends hours each day reading national and international newspapers online. "I'm constantly thinking," she says. Rachel also continues to make art. No longer able to stand for long stretches of time in front of an easel, she's learned how to produce digital art on her computer.

Time spent with family and friends is another key feature of Rachel's life. She cherishes her relationships with her son and in-laws, her neighbors and friends. Rachel says plenty of visitors come to see her. "As a matter of fact," she says, laughing, "I have too many visitors!"

Many of Rachel's friendships developed through her volunteering efforts. She has a special place in her heart for music, and over the years she served on committees for the local opera as well as other music and arts organizations. In addition, she's volunteered for and donated to organizations that support orphans and children in need, as well as individuals who are sick or underprivileged. She says giving of herself in this way not only connected her to many wonderful people but made her life much richer.

Rachel celebrated her latest birthday with a small gathering of close family, friends and neighbors.

Is it luck or good life choices? Is it possible to keep our bodies from wearing down and becoming susceptible to disease? Can more of us enjoy good health and vitality into our 90s or 100s?

Healthy aging doesn't happen by accident. It isn't simply a roll of the dice. How we experience aging is a choice.

Clearly, we're all beholden to some extent to the genes we've inherited. However, genes play a smaller role in overall health than you may think. More often, the life a person leads in their later years is a culmination of personal attitudes, decisions made and actions taken beginning in young adulthood. In other words, you control what can be the most enjoyable and meaningful years of your life.

As scientists broaden our knowledge and understanding of aging and how to add health to our years, now is the perfect time to take stock of your physical and personal well-being. No matter what your age, it's never too late to change the course of your future health!

YOU'RE AGING *RIGHT NOW*

Most babies are born in good health, and unless you developed a childhood illness, chances are you reached young adulthood with relatively few trips to the doctor. What you may not know is that from the moment you were born, your body has been experiencing diverse forms of wear and tear that are at the root of aging. Some scientists believe that the wheels of time start turning even before birth!

During childhood our bodies grow, develop and mature. At the same time, they're aging. Aging is a natural process that begins long before you notice its effects — years before you experience aches and pains; decades before your hair starts taking on tinges of gray; close to a lifetime before you find yourself forgetting where you put your car keys or struggling to remember familiar names.

This is why no matter where you are in life, it's never too early to think about how you want to age and ways you might affect your own aging process.

In this book, we provide you with a commonsense approach to longevity — practical approaches to preserve your health and to maintain vitality through-out your life. But first, it's important to understand how and why aging occurs and what researchers are finding in their efforts to harness harmful forces that often lead to disease and frailty.

HOW LONG WILL YOU LIVE?

Because longer life spans run in some families, it was once commonly believed that your longevity — the length and duration of your life — was determined solely by your genetics. But researchers have found that's not the case. In fact, a study of 400 million people concluded just the opposite — that longevity isn't a matter of genes. Researchers traced the family history for each participant, including dates of birth, causes of death, places lived and family ties. This research and another study published around the same time confirmed that genes play only a small role in a long life.

What researchers are discovering is that your genes interact with several other factors that influence your life and your health. Your lifestyle and the environment in which you live are more influential in determining your life span.

Genetics

Research suggests that only about 15% to 25% of aging is dependent on your genes. But which genes play crucial roles in determining how long you'll live, and how they contribute to longevity, isn't well understood.

Dozens of genes have been shown to influence life span, but so far only a few genes — APOE, FOXO3A and CETP, which protects against cardiovascular disease — consistently show up in most longevity studies. All humans carry these specific genes, but there are different versions (variants) of the genes that influence the behavior of resulting proteins associated with better or worse health. And not all long-lived individuals carry the same variants. What this means is that multiple genes likely play a role or have some type of influence in determining life expectancy. It's not just a few genes that control your future.

Of the genes that have been linked to longevity, some are involved with basic maintenance and function of the body's cells, including DNA repair, chromosome preservation and protection against damage from cells called free radicals (see page 12). Other genes are associated with blood fat (lipid) levels, regulation of inflammation and other processes that reduce the risk of heart disease, stroke and insulin resistance associated with diabetes.

Beyond your genes

While your genes are important, and certain genes may be more protective than others, your genes aren't the only ingredient determining how long and how well you'll live. They respond to and work with whatever else you add to your recipe for daily living.
- **Lifestyle.** Unhealthy habits — a poor diet, inactivity, obesity, high levels of

stress, smoking and alcohol use —
generally result in poorer health, an
increased risk for early-onset illness
and premature death.

- **Environment.** Unhealthy living
conditions; limited access to healthy
foods; exposure to air pollution,
chemicals and toxins; and inadequate
access to health care impact aging and
reduce longevity.
- **Life circumstances.** Lack of social
support, lower socioeconomic status
and education levels can influence
how long and how well people live.
- **Sex.** In every country in the world,
there's a general observation that
individuals born female outlive
individuals born male.

The good news is that many of these
factors are within your control. While
you cannot change the genes you
inherited, what you do with them is up
to you. Your daily actions, or inactions,
may have greater implications than you
realize.

What we're learning from centenarians

Over the past few decades, scientists
have been studying people in their 90s
and 100s to determine what contributes
to their long lives. Individuals who reach
age 100 are known as centenarians.

Those who reach 110 or older are often
referred to as supercentenarians.

To date, what researchers are finding is
that long-lived individuals often have
little in common with one another in
regard to education, income or profes-
sion. The similarities they do share,
however, reflect their lifestyles — many
are nonsmokers, they have a healthy
body weight, they're socially well
connected and they're able to effectively
manage stress.

Data also suggests that for a person's
first seven or eight decades — into your
70s and 80s — lifestyle is a stronger
determinant of health and longevity
than genetics. Factors such as a healthy
diet, avoiding tobacco and staying
physically and socially active are what
enable most individuals to reach a
healthy old age. Genetics appear to play
a progressively important role as you
enter your 80s and beyond.

AGING IS A COMPLEX PROCESS

As scientists delve into the intricacies of
longevity, they're getting a better grasp
on the nitty-gritty details of aging —
what happens at the molecular and
cellular levels. With this knowledge, they
— and the rest of us — are hoping to

gain insights into how we can delay and minimize the effects of aging, whether through lifestyle modifications, drugs or other processes.

Cellular breakdown

The human body is a marvel of microscopic engineering, composed of trillions of cells that keep everything within it working smoothly. How these cells function — and how well they function — generally evolves over time. Aging is what happens when cells begin to change, deteriorate or work less efficiently. This can happen at any point in life.

Changes within cells are what cause our skin to thin and wrinkle, our eyesight to lose its sharpness and our muscles to stiffen. Cellular breakdown also affects how well our body's organs and organ systems perform. For example, a 70-year-old, even one in good health, has about half the lung function and kidney function a young adult has.

As we get older, it's small, long-term changes within and between certain cells that lead to chronic illnesses such as heart disease, high blood pressure, chronic obstructive pulmonary disease (COPD), diabetes and dementia — dis-

eases that can strip us of our vitality and eventually our lives. How quickly or how slowly certain cells break down predicts what diseases we may develop and, more broadly, how long we'll live.

So, while disease can drive aging and loss of life, age itself is a major risk factor for disease and frailty. Geroscience is a field of study that aims to understand how aging occurs and the major role it plays in chronic illness and loss of health.

Other processes at play

Aging involves several forces — actions within our bodies and environmental influences outside them. While there's still much that we don't know about why one individual ages relatively well and another has more difficulty, scientists and researchers are consistently gaining ground in their understanding of the fundamental biology of aging.

Some approaches to aging follow the line of thinking that cellular damage over time leads to the loss of normal functioning and the development of aging. Others are based on the idea that aging follows a programmed timetable — it has an upper limit. No single theory or phenomenon appears to completely explain why aging occurs.

Researchers generally view aging as many processes that interact with and impact each other. Here are some of the biological processes that appear to be at play.

Genetic damage

One hallmark of aging that researchers readily agree on is genetic damage that occurs over time within the body's cells. For many reasons, DNA, the body's intricate blueprint for performing all of its functions, gradually becomes damaged. The body has several ways to repair DNA, but as the damage accumulates, genes, proteins and cells may malfunction, leading to disease and deterioration.

DNA damage can result from forces both within and outside the body. Sometimes, for example, when cells divide and multiply, errors occur in the DNA replication process within a cell and these changes are carried on to new cells, throwing off cellular function and communication within cells.

DNA damage can be especially impactful when it affects stem cells — the precursor cells that give rise to new, specialized cells for the regeneration of skin, digestive, brain and other organ tissues. Genetic damage in stem cells can cause them to stop functioning correctly and make tissue regeneration difficult.

Oxidative stress is another source of DNA damage. It results when cellular structures called mitochondria become damaged. Mitochondria are the cell's powerhouses. They convert food into energy used by cells. During the conversion process, mitochondria produce unstable molecules called reactive oxygen species, better known as free radicals.

Usually, free radicals are kept in check by compounds called antioxidants, which can come from dietary nutrients such as vitamin E, vitamin A and beta carotene. However, lifestyle factors such as smoking, alcohol use, and an unhealthy diet can damage mitochondria and accelerate the production of free radicals, causing oxidative stress.

One of the effects of oxidative stress is deterioration of the endcaps of chromosomes (telomeres). Shortened telomeres are a key feature of aging cells. Telomeres typically get shorter each time a cell divides, but evidence suggests that oxidative stress may also play a role in this particular form of DNA damage.

External factors that can result in genetic damage include sun exposure, which harms skin cell DNA, and polluted air, which damages the DNA of lung cells. These forces can cause chemical alterations that interfere with the way genetic instructions are carried out, ultimately leading to the production of unhealthy cells that contribute to diseases such as skin cancer and lung disease.

Cellular clutter and decline

Your body's genes encode proteins, converting them into forms that allow them to become the basic building blocks of all cells. Proteins can be expressed in many ways, which is why liver cells differ from heart cells — each has their unique function.

Protein regulation is an important part of cell maintenance. Autophagy is the name for the process your body uses to get rid of damaged or redundant cell proteins and parts. When this process doesn't work as it should, cells can get cluttered with wonky proteins, which can affect DNA repair and normal cellular responses. Protein clutter or buildup is seen in age-related conditions such as Alzheimer's disease, which is characterized by clumps of harmful beta-amyloid proteins.

Not only can cells become cluttered with proteins, but their internal structures may become altered. The "skeleton" of a cell (cytoskeleton) is made up of a microscopic network of protein filaments and tubules. Over time, this network becomes more rigid and fixed, so that a cell can't flex and move as it once did, reducing intracellular communication and increasing risk of disease. For example, hardening of the cells that line your blood vessels can impede healthy blood flow and lead to high blood pressure.

Cellular senescence

Research suggests that when some cells within the body deteriorate — whether because of genetic damage, telomere erosion, oxidative stress, protein clutter or other reasons — the cells eventually stop dividing and enter what's called a senescent state. Senescent cells aren't dead, but they aren't functioning appropriately, either. The cells are sometimes described as "Zombie cells."

The body naturally removes many senescent cells but not all. Some linger

Over the last century our life span has nearly doubled. Americans born in the early 1900s had an average life span of just over 45 years. A person born today can reasonably expect to live close to 80 years on average. Unfortunately, our health span hasn't kept pace.

Life span is the number of years of life. Health span is the period of life spent in good health, free from chronic disease and the disabilities of aging. While people are generally living longer today, for many the last decade of life is often racked with chronic age-related diseases that diminish quality of life.

The gap between our average life span and our average health span is now more than a decade and widening.

Researchers at Mayo Clinic and elsewhere are looking for ways to narrow the life span/health span gap so that your final years can be lived to the fullest. The answer is likely multifaceted, including therapies to counter the effects of aging, growth of new medical fields such as regenerative medicine, and continued public health efforts to address unhealthy behaviors that contribute to chronic illness.

Regenerative medicine is a new area of treatment that's shifting emphasis from fighting disease to rebuilding health. Regenerative interventions on the horizon show promise for addressing chronic diseases such as cancer, heart disease and diabetes.

But medical advances and technology can only do so much. The good news is that quite a bit of the aging process is within our own control. Efforts to adopt healthy lifelong habits, for example, are key to ensuring living not just longer, but better.

Graph on opposite page based on Centers for Disease Control and Prevention, American Heart Association and other sources.

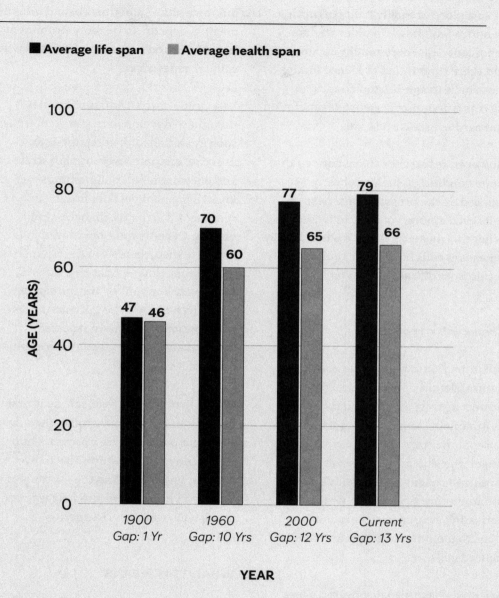

■ Average life span   ■ Average health span

AGE (YEARS)

100

80 — 77 — 79

70 — 65 — 66

60

47 — 46

40

20

0

1900   1960   2000   Current
Gap: 1 Yr Gap: 10 Yrs Gap: 12 Yrs Gap: 13 Yrs

YEAR

and may harm neighboring cells — similar to a piece of moldy fruit corrupting an entire fruit bowl. In older adults, senescent cells more readily accumulate and there's mounting evidence linking these cells to age-related conditions such as osteoporosis, neurodegeneration and cardiovascular disease.

However, researchers have noticed that some conditions, such as obesity, are marked by the presence of senescent cells even among younger individuals. What this means is that it's possible that senescent cells both contribute to and result from disease and aging.

Chronic inflammation

Inflammation is part of the body's natural defense process, designed to protect against external factors such as infections, toxins and trauma and to repair damage. When you cut your finger, the skin around the cut may swell and redden. That's your body's inflammatory response at work, activating a cascade of immune reactions that eliminate germs and repair injured cells.

Scientists have also discovered a less healing inflammatory response — a low-grade inflammation present throughout the body. This form of inflammation, sometimes called inflammaging, appears to be more prominent later in life and is closely associated with cellular senescence.

Low-grade chronic inflammation is thought to develop in response to things such as an unhealthy diet, too little exercise, ongoing levels of high stress and environmental pollutants, as well as underlying medical conditions, such as rheumatoid arthritis, diabetes and obesity. Chronic inflammation also is linked to disturbances in the balance of microorganisms — bacteria, viruses, fungi — that populate the human gut (gut microbiome). The gut microbiome and how it affects many aspects of human health and longevity are ongoing areas of investigation.

From what you just read, it's clear that researchers know more today than ever before about the aging process. Though there's no manual yet for how to live forever, understanding the mechanics of aging can provide links to new ways of living well, well into old age.

WHAT IT ALL MEANS

So, what should you make of all this information?

First off, understand that aging begins very early in life. It's never too early to take steps to protect your well-being in your later years. At the same time, know that it's also never too late to change the course of your health. Among individuals in middle age and older, adopting healthier lifestyles has been found to extend survival, even for people with chronic illnesses.

Second, and most important, don't sell yourself short. Small changes can bring big rewards. You really have the power to alter the course of your later years, allowing you to live longer and in better health. Making healthy choices in your daily life can play a huge role in keeping your body systems in balance and healthy.

Keep in mind that healthy aging doesn't necessarily mean living without disease or being completely absent of illness. To be healthy in old age doesn't mean you have to be superhuman. Healthy aging is about living as well as possible to reduce your risk of cumulative health problems and about feeling as good as possible so that you can enjoy life despite some limitations.

The pages that follow provide you with valuable information and guidance for how to live well throughout your life.

Part 1 takes a look at individual body systems, common patterns of aging within those systems, and steps that may alter those events. In Part 2, you'll have a chance to assess your current well-being and develop a plan for adding health, purpose, independence and years to your life.

Common age-related changes and what you can do

2

Your brain

Upon retirement from his longtime newspaper career, *New York Times* columnist William Safire joined a philanthropic organization dedicated to advancing and sharing interests in science, health and medicine. Safire wrote in his last editorial that he wanted to keep his "synapses snapping" in his later years. And he encouraged his readers to keep active and stay involved.

Increasing evidence suggests that the phrase "Use it or lose it" may apply to the body's most integrated and complex organ — the brain. With age, you may experience some change in your mental abilities. But studies also suggest that you may be able to delay or prevent age-related declines by caring for your overall health and implementing strategies to enhance brain function.

Your later years present an opportunity to do the things you've always wanted — to explore, pursue long-awaited interests and seek new challenges. Steps you take throughout your life that encourage brain health can help you fully enjoy this "golden" time in your life. Lifestyle choices, physical and cognitive activities, and social engagement and support all play a role in reducing cognitive decline.

BRAIN HEALTH

No two people age in the same way. There are older adults who live into their 90s with their memory intact and still able to function as they did in their 60s or 70s. Most individuals, however, experience at least some subtle changes in memory and mental capacity with time.

Your mental strengths and weaknesses as a young adult may be an indicator of your mental skills in your later years. If you've always been good at remembering people's names, you're likely to maintain this skill. If, on the other hand, you have trouble with names, you might not get much better at it with age, unless you make a concentrated effort to improve this skill. It's important to remember that even in your later years, you can still learn and take on new challenges.

To understand brain changes that often occur with age, it's helpful to have some basic knowledge of how the brain works and how it evolves over time.

Neurons and neuroplasticity

The human brain is composed of billions of nerve cells (neurons) and trillions of electrical circuits that connect them. Neurons collect, process and send messages to one another. Tiny gaps between nerve cells (synapses) make it possible for electrical impulses to pass from one nerve cell to the next — connecting neurons in your brain to one another and to neurons in your spinal cord and peripheral nerves. The nervous system is how your brain communicates with other parts of your body.

With age, the number of neurons decreases, resulting in less communication between your brain and the rest of your body. As this happens, your brain actually shrinks in size. This decrease in volume affects specific structures within the brain. Those parts of the brain responsible for cognitive function — our ability to learn, think, reason, remember and make decisions — may diminish more than others. It's why you may feel that your brain isn't as sharp and nimble as it once was.

The good news is, while some of your brain's neurons are lost with age, new connections are made in remaining cells, and new nerve cells may form in other parts of the brain, even in older age. This ability of the brain to modify, change and adapt in both structure and function throughout life is known as neuroplasticity.

Not that long ago, popular thinking was that the brain contained a set number of neurons, that these neurons couldn't be altered, and that with age not much good happened to the brain — neural connections diminished, the size of the brain decreased, and illnesses such as Alzheimer's disease set in. However, research in the last 10 or 15 years has shown that the brain isn't static. On the contrary, it has a great deal of capacity to adapt.

This capacity for neuroplasticity means that you can retrain your brain — to be more attentive to the world around you, to open yourself up to new ways of thinking, and to learn.

COMMON AGE-RELATED CHANGES

For most adults, brain function remains stable throughout life. However, as you get older it may take you longer to perform some tasks than when you were younger. Changes that typically happen with age include the following.

Processing speed

The speed at which you process information and provide a response, such as making a movement or giving an answer to a question, slows a bit with age.

According to some estimates, an older adult's response time is about 1½ times slower than that of a younger adult. What this means is that you may need more time to solve a complex problem than you did in your 30s. Or you may need a little more time and a bit more instruction to master new skills. But when given enough time, older adults are able to come up with accurate, effective solutions equal to those of younger adults.

Memory

Memory is a broad term that describes the ability to remember information. With typical aging, older adults are generally good at retaining information and memories, such as details about a family wedding or a child's graduation. It may just take longer to retrieve this information. The ability to perform well-learned procedures such as riding a bike remains stable. This is an example of what's called procedural memory. Where older adults may notice changes is in working memory, which is the ability to temporarily hold on to information, such as hearing a new phone number and remembering it long enough to call it. Recent memory and the formation of new memories are more vulnerable to aging.

Attention

Attention is the ability to focus on something in order to process information. Simple or focused attention, such as being able to watch and pay attention to a TV program, is generally preserved in older age. But it may be more difficult to do things that divide attention, such as watching TV and talking on the phone at the same time.

The brain can process only so much information at one time. With age, it can become easier to lose focus in a busy environment. However, aging doesn't seem to affect the ability to focus on simple tasks.

Language

Language skills describe how well you can understand and use language, whether it's written or spoken. Older adults retain their vocabulary and their ability to understand written language. But understanding speech can get more difficult with age, especially in someone with hearing problems. It may take more time to find or retrieve a word. However, using a rich vocabulary and engaging in interesting conversation can help you maintain, and possibly even improve, your language skills.

Executive function

Executive function is a term that describes your mental agility. It includes the complex processes that make it possible for you to organize tasks, remember details, think abstractly, manage time and solve problems. These skills generally decline with age. But this doesn't mean that use of such skills isn't possible when you're older; it may just take you longer to engage them than when you were younger.

Emotional processing

Emotional processing is your ability to regulate your emotions so that you can respond appropriately, especially in negative situations. Research shows that older adults generally tend to react less to and recover more easily from negative situations. Older adults also tend to focus on and remember more positive than negative information.

Judgment

Unlike most other aspects of aging, judgment often gets better with age. This is presumably due to crystallized intelligence, knowledge and skills that take experience and time to develop. It's likely why older adults are often viewed as wise sages.

Responsiveness

Age-related changes can occur in the peripheral nerves, those nerves that extend out from your spinal cord. Your peripheral nerves can become weaker and less responsive, influencing both incoming sensory and outgoing motor signals. Sensory changes can affect your perception of temperature and touch. Because each of your muscles is paired with a nerve, motor changes can affect your reaction speed, which also tends to slow over time. That's why you may find it more difficult to catch a ball, stand on a surfboard or avoid a fall.

So, given what you just read, would you consider the fact that it takes you a bit longer to recall the name of a person you rarely see normal? What about forgetting to pick up the dry cleaning? Brain function naturally changes with age, and not all changes are indications of disease. Don't worry if you can't grasp instructions on how to install a new home gadget or computer-related program as quickly as you once did. It's normal.

Also, don't let this information get you down. Sure, your brain's processing speed may not be as robust as it once was, but as an older adult, you've gained certain skills to help offset many age-related declines. With age comes wisdom and valuable life experiences, lessons and insights. Studies also show improvements in certain capacities with age, such as executive function and attention.

CONDITIONS THAT AREN'T TYPICAL

Not all changes that occur later in life are expected. Some people experience a sustained decline in their cognitive health that may involve trouble processing information, frequent confusion, difficulty expressing ideas and even personality changes. These signs and symptoms aren't part of typical aging.

The brain disease most commonly associated with abnormal aging is dementia. Alzheimer's disease is its most common form.

Dementia

Chances are you've wandered around the house looking for your cellphone, and maybe you've driven to the grocery store without your grocery list. After such an event, you may wonder if you're developing dementia. Keep in mind that everyone, regardless of age, has daily memory lapses like this. The difficulties with memory and thinking associated with dementia go beyond simple forgetfulness. Dementia-related difficulties impact a person's ability to perform daily tasks such as managing finances, doing household chores and participating in favorite activities.

Several factors increase the risk of dementia, including age, family history and genetics, cardiovascular problems, diabetes and other health issues.

Much research is being done into the causes of dementia and its progression. Scientists hope one day to be able to spot patterns of cognitive change associated with dementia at the earliest stages to better understand exactly what triggers the disease. Such information could possibly lead to earlier intervention — the initiation of treatment sooner, when it's likely to be most beneficial.

Scientists also hope to better understand how fast or how far people may shift from normal functioning to dementia. For example, why is it that some peoples' memories stabilize after only mild memory loss, while others' memories and other cognitive functions continue to decline quickly?

Alzheimer's disease

Alzheimer's disease is the most common form of dementia and is diagnosed when healthy brain tissue progressively degenerates, leading to irreversible mental impairment. Most people with Alzheimer's disease share certain signs and symptoms. They include:

- A gradual loss of memory for recent events and an inability to process new information.
- A progressive tendency to repeat oneself, misplace objects, become confused and get lost.
- A gradual disintegration of personality and judgment.
- Increasing irritability, anxiety, depression, confusion and restlessness.

As the disease progresses, these signs and symptoms become more serious and more noticeable, often over a period of years.

The exact causes of Alzheimer's disease aren't fully understood. Scientists believe that for most people, it results from a combination of genetic, lifestyle and environmental factors that affect the brain over time. Risk tends to be higher in people of Black and Asian ancestry and other ethnic groups.

A 2021 study found that Native Hawaiians and descendants of Pacific Islanders show a higher proportion of Alzheimer's disease than the rest of the U.S. population and are diagnosed at a younger age.

Rarely, Alzheimer's disease is triggered by specific genetic changes that virtually guarantee a person will develop the disease. These rare occurrences usually result in onset of the disease in middle age.

Brain changes associated with Alzheimer's disease most often start in the region that controls memory, but the process begins years before the first symptoms. The loss of neurons spreads in a somewhat predictable pattern to other regions of the brain. By the late stage of the disease, the brain has degenerated significantly.

Researchers hoping to better understand the cause of Alzheimer's disease are focused on the role of two proteins:

- **Plaques.** Beta-amyloid is a fragment of a larger protein. When these fragments cluster together, they appear to have a toxic effect on neurons and to disrupt cell-to-cell communication. These clusters form larger deposits called amyloid plaques, which also include other cellular debris.
- **Tangles.** Tau proteins play a part in a neuron's internal support and the transport system to carry nutrients and other essential materials. In Alzheimer's disease, tau proteins change shape and organize themselves into structures called neurofibrillary tangles. The tangles disrupt the transport system and are toxic to cells.

Alzheimer's disease isn't inevitable, even if you're at risk. And not all individuals with characteristics of Alzheimer's display its signs and symptoms. In one study, researchers who followed nearly 700 Catholic nuns for several years found that when the brains of several nuns were examined, they contained plaques and tangles. However, the nuns displayed no clinical evidence of dementia.

Although there's no cure for Alzheimer's disease or a surefire way to prevent it, scientists continue to make progress in understanding it. Doctors are able to diagnose the condition at much earlier stages than in decades past.

And while there aren't any definitive treatments for the disease, some therapies are available that can help improve quality of life for people who have it. New drugs are being studied, and scientists have discovered several gene variants associated with Alzheimer's disease, which may lead to new treatments to help block its progression.

BUILDING YOUR COGNITIVE RESERVE

If you were told that you had specific changes in your brain, such as shrinkage in key regions associated with memory, and that these changes are often seen in someone with dementia, chances are you'd think the worst. But not everyone who experiences dementia-related brain changes shows signs of the disease. Why is this?

Two people can have similar amounts of the hallmark plaques and tangles of Alzheimer's disease. Yet, one may have debilitating symptoms while the other has no issues with memory at all. Experts think that the difference between the two comes down to what's called cognitive reserve. Simply put, cognitive reserve is how well your brain is able to cope with — or adjust to — pathological changes, such as those associated with dementia.

Experts believe that an individual's cognitive reserve capacity isn't determined at birth. It may develop and expand throughout life; possibly offsetting some of the brain changes that lead to dementia. Certain activities are thought to help develop more cognitive reserve. Those activities that are at least moderately challenging to the brain, such as learning a new skill or a new language, seem to help most in building this reserve.

Whether or not you're born with a good cognitive reserve, you can build it through education and activities such as reading, playing an instrument and practicing mindfulness. It seems that people who spend more time engaged in learning throughout their lives develop more robust networks of neurons in their brains and bolster the connections between them.

A strong network of neurons may be a powerful tool in combating cell damage that leads to dementia.

YOUR MENTAL AND EMOTIONAL WELL-BEING

Brain (cognitive) health is about more than just maintaining good memory. Mental and emotional well-being are other important aspects of aging. Life events and transitions that occur in peoples' later years can lead to conditions such as anxiety and depression. The good news, though, is that many people find their mental and emotional well-being actually improves with age.

A study by research psychologists at Stanford University who observed

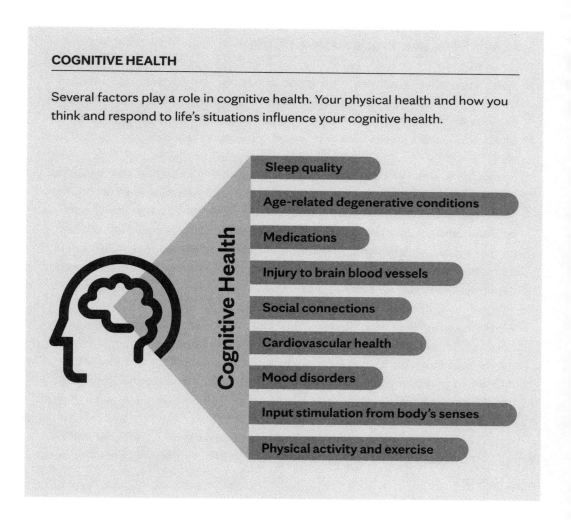

COGNITIVE HEALTH

Several factors play a role in cognitive health. Your physical health and how you think and respond to life's situations influence your cognitive health.

Cognitive Health

- Sleep quality
- Age-related degenerative conditions
- Medications
- Injury to brain blood vessels
- Social connections
- Cardiovascular health
- Mood disorders
- Input stimulation from body's senses
- Physical activity and exercise

emotional wellness in a group of people over the course of five and then 10 years found that most reported greater emotional stability as they got older.

Despite having more chronic illnesses, it turns out that individuals often experience a decrease in negative emotions and increase in positive emotions with age. Studies also indicate that older adults tend to experience fewer fluctuations in their emotions, and as a result are generally better able to control their emotions.

HEARING LOSS AND YOUR MENTAL HEALTH

Humans are social creatures — most people seek out connections with others and thrive on them. Living in an intensely social world can be difficult when your ability to communicate is hampered. Hearing loss can strain your relationships with family, friends, coworkers and anyone with whom you interact regularly.

For example, when you can't hear much of what's being said at a dinner party, you may tire quickly or feel left out. This may cause you to skip these events and stay home. At the store, you may have trouble hearing your total charge from a soft-spoken cashier. If your partner is talking to you while you're working in front of a running faucet or dishwasher, you may not understand what's being said. Other factors associated with hearing loss, such as social isolation, low self-esteem and depression, may further strain relationships.

When you struggle to hear, conversations can quickly become frustrating and tiresome. Although you want to spend time with your family and friends, interacting may get too stressful. It's natural to try to avoid situations that you know will be difficult. In so doing, you may cut yourself off from the world around you and the people who love you.

If you've been living with hearing loss for any amount of time, it probably won't surprise you to learn that researchers have uncovered links between hearing impair-

Research suggests that individual personality traits also tend to remain stable over time. So, for instance, if you're outgoing in your 40s and 50s, it's a good bet that you'll continue to be an outgoing person in your 60s, 70s and beyond.

Life triggers

Chances are you've already taken steps to plan for your financial stability in your older years. What about your emotional stability? It's also important to invest in your emotional well-being. Often this

ment and depression and anxiety. If you can't hear well, you may avoid being around other people. This self-imposed isolation can lead to loneliness, which in turn leads to depression.

There's a lot of new research pointing to the connection between emotional well-being and untreated hearing impairment. One study by researchers at Johns Hopkins University found that people who don't address hearing loss in middle age are more at risk for developing dementia.

The science behind this risk is that hearing impairment affects our brain's ability to encode and remember information. If you can't hear what's being said, then you can't encode and remember it as well. It may also be the case that struggling to hear requires a lot more cognitive energy, so it makes it more challenging for your brain to create new memories. In fact, in older adults with normal cognitive function, hearing loss is predictive of later cognitive decline.

This is part of the reason why preserving your hearing is very important. If you have diminished hearing, work with an audiologist to see if you need hearing aids and to learn tips to help you hear better. You can read more about hearing loss in the next chapter.

means examining and preparing for the life triggers that could impact your emotional health.

Along with a list of things that you look forward to in retirement, make a list of things that concern or worry you. This may include physical events, such as developing a disease or problems with your hearing or eyesight. Other life triggers may include leaving a beloved career, losing your spouse or a close friend or family member, or your chil-dren leaving the house. Major transitions can lead to difficult emotions and illness such as depression.

If you know that you may face a difficult event, strategize now for how you'll handle it. For example, if you plan to retire soon, how will you keep busy? If you're moving to a new community, how will you meet people and get involved? If a parent is having health issues, how can you divide your time between your parent and your own family?

COPING WITH GRIEF AND LOSS

Grief and loss are inevitable parts of aging that can impact all areas of your life, including your job and your relationships with friends and family. While there can be an overlap between grief and depression, grief isn't depression. Sadness associated with grief typically decreases with time.

Everyone reacts to and copes differently with death. Grieving and embracing the time you spent with a loved one are important processes to help you face the most acute stages of grief. It may take months to a year to come to terms with such a loss, and there's no deadline for when grief should end. But research supports the idea that most people can recover from the death of a loved one on their own with time if they have social support and practice healthy habits. Avoiding your feelings and isolating yourself disrupt the healing process.

While the loss of a spouse or close friend can trigger intense sadness, there are ways to enhance your resilience, which can help you cope during more difficult times.

Stress

One of the biggest culprits preventing healthy aging is one you may not expect: stress. Stress doesn't go away with age. Increasingly, researchers are viewing stress — how much we face and how well we deal with it — as a critical factor in how well we age.

Stress occurs when the demands in your life exceed your ability to cope with them. Many things can cause stress, from simple things, such as having to stand in line for a long time at the checkout counter, to more serious challenges, such as losing your job or developing an illness.

Whatever the cause of your stress, if it's overwhelming you, you need to address it. Stress is a serious health risk. When you experience stress, your heart beats faster, your blood pressure rises and your breathing may quicken. If stressful situations pile up one after another, your

Accept your feelings. Know that feelings of grief are normal and you might experience a wide range of emotions, including sadness, anger or exhaustion. If you're feeling overwhelmed, talk to a grief therapist, who can help you cope with those feelings.

Take care of yourself. Grieving can take a physical toll. Focusing on eating healthy foods, exercising and getting plenty of sleep can support both your physical and emotional health.

Stay socially connected. This is one of the most important ways to avoid depression in general, but especially after experiencing the loss of a loved one. During difficult times, try to maintain social connections, whether this means getting together with close friends, joining a book club, having a poker night, or being part of a faith-based community.

body has no chance to recover, making you more vulnerable to long-term health problems.

Stressful life events can trigger depression, and they may also worsen the signs and symptoms of other mental health disorders, such as anxiety.

Studies consistently show that people who do best at managing stress, who tend to be more resilient to life's challenges, also tend to stay the healthiest in older age. Dealing with stress is a critical part of both your physical and your emotional health. If you don't consider yourself a very resilient person, there are skills you can develop to help you remain positive and cope more easily with life's challenging experiences (see page 182).

Depression

Depression is a serious mood disorder. It can affect the way you feel, act and think. Depression is common in older adults, but it isn't a normal part of aging. In fact, studies show that most older adults feel satisfied with their lives, despite having more illnesses or physical ailments than younger individuals.

There's no single cause of depression. Experts believe a genetic vulnerability to

the disease combined with environmental factors, such as stress or physical illness, may trigger an imbalance in brain chemicals called neurotransmitters. Imbalances in three neurotransmitters — serotonin, norepinephrine and dopamine — seem to be linked to depression.

The hallmark symptoms of the disease are a depressed mood and loss of interest in activities that were once enjoyed. Other signs and symptoms may include sleep disturbances, such as early awakening, sleeping too much or having trouble falling asleep; decreased concentration, attention and memory; changes in appetite and unexplained weight gain or loss; restlessness, agitation or irritability; and feelings of helplessness, worthlessness or guilt. Depression can also cause a wide variety of physical complaints, such as fatigue, headache, digestive problems and chronic pain.

A number of events and conditions appear to increase a person's likelihood of becoming depressed. In many cases, depression results from not just one risk factor but a combination of them. These include a family history of depression; stressful life events, such as the loss of a loved one or a divorce; deeply upsetting past experiences, such as childhood abuse; dependence on drugs or alcohol;

other mental health issues, such as an anxiety or eating disorder; and certain personality traits, such as being overly self-critical or pessimistic or easily overwhelmed.

If you feel that you may be depressed, it's important to seek help from your health care provider. Antidepressant medications are often the first line of treatment. Another common treatment is psychotherapy, also called talk therapy or counseling. The most effective treatment for depression is often the combination of medication and psycho-therapy.

Excessive alcohol use

Alcoholism and alcohol abuse are less prevalent among older adults than among the general population, but that doesn't mean older adults are immune to them. Among adults who abuse alcohol, one-third develop the problem later in life, perhaps in reaction to retirement, failing health or the death of a spouse.

If you reach for a glass of wine or a bottle of beer to self-soothe, remember that too much alcohol can lead to depression, anxiety and even psychosis and antisocial behavior. It's also import-ant to be aware that with age, your body

can become more sensitive to alcohol. If your drinking habits don't change to compensate for that sensitivity, you could find that you have an alcohol problem.

KEYS TO BRAIN HEALTH

It's never too early to engage in habits that can help offset age-related cognitive changes and enhance your mental well-being. Taking steps now to protect your brain can help it stay healthy as you age. Researchers have found that about a third of the time, dementia is caused by risk factors that you can control. This means, in theory, if you can manage specific aspects of your health, you may be able to reduce your risk of developing brain-related conditions.

Keeping your brain healthy is a lifelong process. Challenging and engaging your brain throughout your lifetime may increase your cognitive reserve and the brain protection it offers (see page 26). Addressing general health issues, such as physical inactivity, high blood pressure, tobacco use, stress and anxiety, has also been shown to be helpful for brain functioning and mental health.

While paying attention to these issues is important at any age, it's especially important in midlife. Caring for your overall health can help protect your blood vessels, for example, which may prevent cognitive decline later in life. Good cardiovascular health is good for not only your heart but also your brain.

Following are more details about what researchers have found to be most helpful in promoting brain health and mental well-being across the life span. Overall, these measures provide a road map for better brain aging.

Keep physically active

In one study, researchers divided participants into two groups. One group took part in aerobic exercise; the other group performed stretching and balance exercises. After one year, researchers noticed that the individuals involved with aerobic exercise had a larger hippocampus — the part of the brain that makes new memories.

In another study, researchers found that people with a gene that causes Alzheimer's disease who exercised for 150 minutes or more each week delayed onset of the disease by several years. People with the gene who exercised less than 150 minutes a week developed Alzheimer's disease more quickly. While it's not certain that exercise can reduce the risk of Alzheimer's disease, this research suggests that it may.

What is it about physical activity that makes it so important? Experts think exercise keeps blood flowing, which is beneficial to brain health. It also boosts the level of chemicals that naturally protect the brain. And physical activity helps make up for the connections between nerve cells in your brain that are lost as you age.

Data indicates that overall mental functioning is less likely to decline in people who are physically active on a regular basis. Physical activity helps provide protection against other diseases that can increase your risk of dementia, including high blood pressure, diabetes and high cholesterol. It may also give your immune system a boost and help combat chronic inflammation. Finally, physical activity helps offset symptoms of stress, anxiety and depression.

Make sleep a priority

It's not news that getting enough good-quality sleep is essential for overall health and well-being. Most people are aware that sleep is important. But in terms of dementia risk, good sleep seems to be especially critical.

Research suggests that not getting enough good sleep over a number of years may increase the risk of dementia. In one analysis, researchers found that people whose sleep is interrupted over many years are more at risk of developing dementia. Researchers also have found that individuals who don't get enough sleep may be twice as likely to develop Alzheimer's disease.

Why is sleep so important? Earlier, we learned that clumps of the protein beta-amyloid harden into plaques. These plaques cause nerve cells in the brain to die. This process is thought to lead to Alzheimer's disease. During sleep, beta-amyloid and other toxins are cleared from the brain. If you don't get good sleep, especially over a long period of time, this process may not work as well. Lack of sleep can increase risk of dementia in other ways, too. (Poor sleep can also increase your risk of other diseases such as high blood pressure and diabetes.)

Adequate sleep is critical to your mental health. Poor sleep can exacerbate symptoms of depression, stress and anxiety. For all these reasons, addressing sleep issues and improving sleep are important to brain health. You can read more about ways to improve sleep in Chapter 9.

Stay socially engaged

People who have many social contacts and regularly engage with other people may be half as likely to experience memory problems. How many people are part of your social network, how diverse your connections are and how often you're in touch with the people in your social circle all play a role in how well your brain functions. That makes staying connected with others, especially later in life, an important factor in preserving brain health and preventing brain changes that can lead to dementia.

Social connections are thought to benefit the brain in many ways. Research suggests that engaging with others triggers the release of chemicals such as serotonin and dopamine, which improve mood and outlook and protect the brain from dementia, especially dementia caused by Alzheimer's disease. Social connections are thought to boost a person's cognitive reserve, which helps buoy the brain against age-related changes. In addition, people who have larger social networks and spend more time engaged with the people in them perform better in thinking skills. You can read more about the benefits of social engagement in Chapter 13.

Social isolation, meanwhile, increases the risk that you will have trouble with thinking skills and memory. It also makes Alzheimer's disease more likely. And it may increase the odds of developing conditions linked to Alzheimer's disease, such as high blood pressure and heart disease, as well as increase your risk of depression and other mental health disorders.

Keep stress in check

Several studies show that chronic stress — the feeling of constantly being overwhelmed by one or more of life's challenges — can result in shrinkage (atrophy) of an area of the brain known as the hippocampus, important to the creation and storage of memories. High levels of stress and prolonged states of stress can increase chronic inflammation and affect cell aging. Stress is thought to affect the length of telomeres, genetic structures at the end of cell chromosomes.

Stress can affect brain health in other ways. When you're faced with a stressful situation, a surge of hormones temporar-

ily increases your blood pressure and causes your blood vessels to narrow. While there's no proof that stress can cause long-term high blood pressure on its own, it's linked to factors that can increase your risk of having high blood pressure. In times of stress, some people turn to unhealthy habits such as smoking, drinking too much alcohol and eating unhealthy foods, all of which can lead to high blood pressure.

Reducing stress can help you to become a more productive and happier person. As you learn how to relax and manage stress, you may even find yourself enjoying things that once seemed burdensome. Just as important, letting go of stress can often improve your mental health.

There are several strategies that can help keep stress in check. They include exercise; mind-body therapies such as deep breathing, meditation and yoga; and simplifying your daily schedule. These practices may also improve overall emotional well-being.

Mind-body therapies are based on the idea that the mind and body are intricately connected and that the mind has the capacity to affect the body. Mind-body practices are discussed in detail in Chapter 16.

Eat brain-friendly foods

Following a mostly plant-based diet, such as the Mediterranean diet or the Mayo Clinic diet, may help prevent dementia. These diets, rich in fruits, vegetables, olive oil, legumes, whole grains and fish, are thought to be good for overall brain health and may also play a role in reducing dementia risk.

Studies have shown that people who follow a Mediterranean diet seem less likely to have Alzheimer's disease than those who don't follow such a diet. Studies also suggest that following a Mediterranean diet may slow mental decline in older adults, keep mild cognitive impairment from progressing to Alzheimer's disease and reduce the risk of mild cognitive impairment.

The foods emphasized in plant-based diets may lower cholesterol and blood sugar, which helps protect blood vessels and, in turn, reduces the risk of stroke and dementia. They may also help prevent the loss of brain tissue associated with Alzheimer's disease.

In particular, dementia researchers have been studying fish, one of the main components of the Mediterranean diet and the Mayo Clinic diet. Some studies suggest that people who carry a version of the apolipoprotein E (APOE) gene — which is linked to a higher Alzheimer's risk — may experience fewer Alzheimer's-related brain changes if they eat seafood on a regular basis.

One area of concern with seafood is its mercury content. Mercury is a toxin, and in high amounts it can harm the brain. However, studies suggest that when eaten in moderate amounts, seafood helps prevent disease-related changes in the brain linked to Alzheimer's disease, even with its higher levels of mercury.

For more information on healthy eating to help prevent aging, see Chapter 15.

Reduce your risk of stroke

The health of your blood vessels is critical to brain health. If your blood vessels weaken or become damaged, they can't get nutrients and oxygen to nerve cells in the brain that need them to function. The following steps can help preserve your blood vessel health.

Don't smoke

When you inhale tobacco smoke, the chemicals quickly travel from your lungs into your blood, reaching every organ in your body and causing inflammation in any tissue they come in contact with. The poisons in tobacco can pose an immediate danger — sudden blood clots, heart attacks and strokes. In addition, neurotoxins found in cigarette smoke may harm the brain and make a stroke more likely.

Manage high blood pressure

High blood pressure weakens the arteries that keep blood flowing through your body. It can cause a stroke, but it can also cause so-called silent strokes that you may not notice. Over time, strokes can cause scarring in the blood vessels. This scarring leads to problems with blood flow in the brain, which can cause problems in how different parts of the brain function. It can also cause parts of the brain to stop working completely.

Manage diabetes

If you have diabetes, you're more likely to have a stroke, in part because diabetes damages blood vessels. This alone makes managing diabetes a key factor in reducing your risk of stroke and, in turn, dementia. Diabetes also has other links to dementia. Excess blood sugar may cause more inflammation in the brain, which can cause problems with how well the brain functions. Plus, developing diabetes late in life also seems to be linked to a higher risk of dementia.

Avoid or limit alcohol

Studies suggest that excessive alcohol consumption — more than two drinks a day — can increase your risk of a stroke as much as does high blood pressure or diabetes. People who consume too much alcohol for years also can experience brain damage as a result of poor nutrition and are at higher risk of developing memory problems and dementia.

Individuals with alcohol use disorder are often malnourished, either because they don't eat enough healthy foods containing essential nutrients or because alcohol and its metabolism prevent the body from properly absorbing, digesting and using those nutrients.

ADDITIONAL TOOLS FOR STAYING MENTALLY SHARP

It's never too early to start developing habits that can help offset age-related memory changes. Here are some practical strategies that can improve your everyday memory and ability to process information. These strategies may also help you keep your brain in shape.

Keep a calendar and a task list

In today's world, you may find yourself bombarded with lots of details from all directions — names, numbers, passwords, to-do lists. If you feel like your brain wasn't designed to lug around this type of information, you're right. When you're trying to track too many tedious details, you're actually more prone to memory lapses. A calendar and organization system can help protect you from information overload.

Have a system

Most of the information you need to remember on your daily to-do list will probably fall into one of the following categories:

- Events that happen at a particular time (such as appointments and meetings).
- Tasks that need to get done, though not at a scheduled time (including doing work tasks and home chores and taking medications).
- Addresses, phone numbers and other contact information for the key people in your life.

Designate a separate section in your cellphone, computer or datebook to track each type of information. It's easier to remember and process information when it's separated according to category, rather than being jumbled together in one big list. You may also benefit from a note-taking area, where you can record events that happen throughout the day, such as information from an important phone call.

Check off tasks when they're complete

Use an X or some other notation. This makes it easier to track unfinished items and leaves no question about whether routine tasks, such as taking medications, were completed. If you think your memory is still sharp enough to skip this step, think again. It's wise to establish this habit early. And you'll likely benefit from a motivating sense of accomplishment as you mark off tasks.

Over time, you'll surely develop your own strategies, shortcuts and abbreviations that make your calendar system work best for you. Experts agree that there isn't one right way to keep a calendar or a list. The best calendar system is just the one that suits your individual needs and takes the least amount of time and energy to maintain.

Clear the clutter

Nowadays, there are whole stores devoted to bins, baskets, cases, containers, hooks and hangers to help you get organized. You don't have to alphabetize every drawer and shelf. But keeping your environment clutter-free can help minimize distractions and improve your memory.

You might start with your mail. It's not easy to wrangle the endless stream of junk mail, bills, bank statements, meeting notices and special announcements that you receive each week. Instead of letting paper accumulate in miscellaneous piles, sort mail and other documents as soon as you get them. As you sort, ask yourself: "Will I ever need this again?" If the answer is yes, keep it. If the answer is no, throw it away.

Have designated locations

Store frequently used items in the same place, whether at work or at home. Carry your car keys or house keys in the same location every time you use them — always in the same pocket or handbag — and always return them to a designated spot when you're finished with them. Keep the kitchen utensils that you use for certain tasks together in convenient locations and put them back in the same spot.

Use a toolbox to store your tools. Always put the tools back when you're done using them so that you know where they are for next time.

Be attentive

Attention happens when you focus on a task, interaction or event. This skill is an important part of memory processing. It takes attention and concentration for information to come into your brain at the beginning of the memory process, so that it can be stored properly and retrieved when you need it. As you age, sustaining attention can be difficult.

To help maintain attention, focus on the present. Before you start a conversation or task, take a few deep breaths. Then look closely at the person or task in front of you. You can also use your senses to help you focus on the present. Thinking about smells or sounds around you can bring awareness of your surroundings and help you concentrate and remember.

To help improve your attention:
- **Minimize distractions.** Turn off the radio or TV while you're reading instructions or having a conversation.

Pull the earbuds out of your ears. Control your work environment to reduce interruptions, such as shutting the office door when you need to concentrate. And what about the chimes, rings and alerts coming from your cellphone or computer? Consider silencing them for a couple of hours each day — or at least while you're working on a project.

- **Perform one task or activity at a time.** Whenever possible, do one thing at a time. Choose to focus for a set period of time and then take a break.
- **Be selective.** Selective attention is the type of attention you rely on when having a conversation in a crowded restaurant. You tune out background noise and other conversations to focus on a select task — in this case, whatever

A WORD ON 'BRAIN TRAINING'

What about formal activities specifically designed to stimulate the mind? There's been some buzz around brain (cognitive) training as a means of helping improve certain brain functions such as memory, language and processing speed. This type of structured program uses repetitive memory and reasoning exercises. They may be computer assisted or done in person, one-on-one or in small groups.

According to researchers, there's not much proof that these activities help. Brain-training products that are widely advertised as a way to give the brain a boost may offer short-term benefits in the specific areas that are addressed, for example, reasoning, decision-making and language. But at this point, no evidence shows that they're helpful beyond the short term or that they can help keep dementia from developing.

Experts say you'll get the most benefit from doing activities that stimulate your brain throughout your life. Getting a good education, working in a mentally stimulating job and taking up mentally engaging pastimes or social activities are all good options.

your dinner companion is saying. You can use this same technique to be selective about what you're trying to remember. When meeting several new people at the same time, for example, try to focus on retaining just a handful of key names — better to remember a few than to be confused about everyone. When reading a news article, pick out a few facts or ideas that may be the most important to remember instead of trying to retain the entire article.

Use memory tricks

Studies suggest that memory techniques can be useful aids. Experiment with the following time-honored tips to see which work best for you. Most prompt you to encode information more efficiently — that is, to mentally focus on information when you first encounter it and to manipulate it in such a way that it helps you remember. Approach memory techniques as if you're playing a game — have fun with them. Being creative (or even outlandish) with these techniques can make them more effective.

Repeat, rehash and revisit

Repeating new information helps you pay attention to it and encode it proper-ly. Try to repeat factual information — such as names and numbers — several times when first trying to learn it. For example, when you meet new people, try to use their names in conversation right away to help you remember them. The same technique works for directions. Repeat directions out loud a few times to properly process the information and order of steps. Similarly, when you want to remember key concepts or ideas, talk about them with others.

Do mental aerobics

One way to keep your mind sharp may simply be exercising it. Just as regular physical activity improves your heart and lung capacity, brain activities may improve your brain function. Brain activities may even help build your cognitive reserve.

Start simple. Spend time each day doing crossword puzzles, number games and everyday tasks that require you to think — mental aerobics to stretch your brain. You might also seek out activities that work different areas of the brain. For example, try jigsaw puzzles to sharpen your spatial-relationship skills. Attend a concert or lecture to hone your sound-processing skills. The list is endless.

Try new things

Lifelong learning and mental stimulation are sure to make life more interesting and enriching. And it's possible these activities may lower your risk of memory decline and Alzheimer's disease.

While you may not be able to do some things as quickly as when you were younger, age shouldn't stop you from pursuing new frontiers. Studies show that older adults learn new skills as well as younger adults do. Younger adults may mentally process information faster, but older adults can apply more wisdom and experience.

Don't be afraid to test your limits. Former president George H. W. Bush celebrated his 75th birthday by skydiving. Artist Georgia O'Keeffe returned to painting and sculpting at the age of 86 and went on to receive the National Medal of Arts. At the age of 88, actress Betty White became the oldest person to guest-host "Saturday Night Live," and she won an Emmy Award for her efforts. Quite simply, it's never too late to turn out some of your best work.

The experience of age provides a rich backdrop for developing skills, embracing change and integrating new knowledge into your life.

3

Your senses

Our five senses — sight, hearing, smell, taste and touch — are detection systems that let us gather information from the world around us, understand our environment and interact with other people. They help us with basic survival, such as being able to communicate, to sense a too-hot surface, and to not eat rotting food. They're also conduits to life's pleasures, from a gourmet dinner and piano concerto to a majestic sunset and the comfort of a soft sweater.

The stimuli our senses receive are sent to the brain, where they're processed to create a complete picture of our surroundings. Our senses are also closely connected to our memories and emotions. And though each of our five sensory systems are separate, they closely collaborate and sometimes even compensate for one another.

With age, each of our senses changes. It's important to understand and anticipate these changes and, when possible, to try to preserve sensory functioning.

Maintaining sensory health is critical not just to protect your safety but so you can continue to enjoy the many wonders and experiences your senses provide.

SIGHT

Most of us start to notice changes to our vision in our early to mid-40s. For the most part, these changes don't cause serious problems and are often easily corrected.

Difficulty reading

It's common to lose the ability to see up close as you age, a condition called presbyopia. With this condition, it becomes more difficult to read fine print, resulting in the need for reading glasses. This happens because our eyes gradually lose their elasticity and ability to change shape, making it more difficult to focus on close-up objects.

Presbyopia generally worsens with age, and by the time you're 65, your lenses have lost most of their elasticity. The condition is most commonly corrected with glasses or contact lenses. Eyedrops or intraocular lens implants placed during cataract surgery may also be an option for some individuals.

Colors and light

You may find that your eyes need more time to adjust to changing light levels, such as going from the bright outdoors to a dark room indoors. And you may have more difficulty distinguishing colors, such as blue from black, as you get older. Factors thought to contribute to greater difficulties with color vision include reduced pupil size, resulting in less light into the eye; increased yellowing of the eye's lens; and alterations in the sensitivity of the vision pathways, all changes that commonly occur as you get older.

Dry eyes

Another noticeable change has to do with how your eyes feel. Tear production tends to decrease as you get older. Decreased production often destabilizes the tear film, creating dry spots on the surface that irritate the eye. Some people produce a normal amount of tears, but their tear fluid is of poor quality and lacks essential components for eye lubrication. Certain medications can also cause dry eyes.

When your tears aren't able to provide adequate lubrication, your eyes may sting, burn or feel scratchy. Dry eyes can also lead to eye fatigue and increased sensitivity to light. Over-the-counter products and medications can help restore normal tear film.

Taking steps to keep your eyes from drying out is important. This includes not letting air blow into your eyes from hair dryers, air conditioners or fans; wearing glasses to protect your eyes from the wind; and keeping the humidity in your home between 30% and 50%. Keep the edges (margins) of your eyelids clean and free of crust, so that the glands can secrete the oils needed to prevent tear film from evaporating.

Floaters

As you get older you may notice the appearance of small spots in your field of vision that move around when you move your eyes. The spots may look like a cobweb or squiggly line. These visual disturbances are known as floaters. Floaters are common and generally increase with age. They tend to be most noticeable in bright sunlight or when looking at a white background.

The internal cavity of your eye is filled with a clear, jellylike substance called the vitreous humor. With age, the consistency of this substance changes and it partially liquifies, which causes it to shrink and pull away from the interior surface of the eye. When this happens, the vitreous humor can become stringy. The floaters that you see in your visual field are actually shadows of the strings cast upon the retina. If you suddenly notice a lot of floaters, you should contact your eye doctor as soon as possible. The problem could be more serious.

Conditions that aren't typical

A number of vision changes naturally occur with age, but certain changes may signal a serious eye disorder. Though common, these conditions shouldn't be considered normal. If left untreated, they could lead to vision loss. The best way to catch these conditions early, when they're most easily treated, is with regular eye exams (see pages 278-279).

Cataracts

A cataract develops from the clouding of your normally clear lens. It's the leading cause of reversible vision loss in the world. With age, almost everyone experiences cataracts to some degree. In the United States, approximately half of all Americans have cataracts by age 80, and millions of cataract surgeries are performed yearly.

It's normal for the lens of your eye to cloud as you get older. It's likely that each of us is on the way to developing a cataract. Most cataracts develop slowly and don't disturb your eyesight early on. By age 80, however, more than half of all Americans either have cataracts or have had surgery to remove them.

How you deal with a cataract will depend on how severe the condition is and how well you tolerate blurred vision. Stronger lighting and eyeglasses can help compensate for vision loss associated with cataracts. But if your vision becomes moderately to significantly impaired and jeopardizes your quality of life, you may need to seek treatment, which involves surgery.

Glaucoma

Glaucoma results from damage to the optic nerve, the bundle of nerve fibers that carry signals between the eye and the brain. Abnormally high pressure inside your eye is usually what damages the optic nerve. As the nerve deteriorates, blind spots develop in your visual field, typically starting with your side (peripheral) vision.

Fortunately, only a small number of people with glaucoma ever lose their sight completely. That's because medical advances have made it easier to detect and treat the disease. If caught early, glaucoma may never cause detectable vision loss. But having glaucoma does require lifelong monitoring and treatment. Medications are the most common treatment for the disease. In some cases, surgery may be necessary.

Macular degeneration

Age-related macular degeneration develops when tissue in the macula — the part of the retina responsible for your central vision — begins to deteriorate. The result is blurred vision or a blind spot in your visual field. The disease tends to develop as you get older, hence the "age-related" part of its name.

Macular degeneration affects your central vision but not your side (peripheral) vision; thus, it doesn't cause total blindness. Still, the loss of clear central vision — critical to many routine tasks, including any type of detail work — greatly affects your independence and quality of life.

Age-related macular degeneration is the leading cause of vision loss in Americans age 60 and older. And as the number of older adults increases, the number of people with macular degeneration is expected to increase. The good news is a handful of therapies can effectively slow the most serious, vision-threatening stages of the disease, and newer treatments in clinical trials are very promising.

Retinal vessel occlusions

Intricate networks of arteries and veins support the eye's retina. They connect to major blood vessels that enter the eye through the optic nerve. Sometimes, these arteries and veins can become blocked, a condition known as retinal vessel occlusion. The condition is common in older adults and can result in reduced vision or vision loss.

Various factors can obstruct a blood vessel. They include a blood clot, the accumulation of fatty deposits (plaques) in the vessel and the collapse of a vessel wall or compression of a wall from outside pressure. The location of the blockage, the presence of swelling and how much time elapses before treatment are key factors in a successful outcome. Several conditions can result from blockage of blood vessels in the retina.

What you can do

Is poor vision inevitable as you grow older? Not necessarily. Everyone's vision changes with age, but there are steps you can take to help protect your eyesight and reduce your risk of some diseases. In addition to regular eye exams, here are steps to prevent vision problems.

Use protective eyewear

One of the most effective ways to protect your vision is to wear safety glasses or goggles in situations that could potentially injure your eyes. This includes at work, at home and at play.

Wear sunglasses

Ultraviolet (UV) rays from the sun can damage your eyes as well as your skin. Long-term exposure to UV radiation can increase your risk of eye disease, particularly cataracts and age-related macular degeneration. Look for sunglasses that block 99% to 100% of ultraviolet A and ultraviolet B light.

Avoid eyestrain

Any type of work or activity that depends on intensive use of your eyes — such as driving, reading, time in front of a computer or on a cellphone or certain activities such as crafts — may cause eyestrain. This doesn't lead to permanent eye damage, but it can affect your everyday vision. Signs and symptoms of eyestrain include eye fatigue, blurry or double vision, headaches, neck or back pain, squinting and sensitivity to light.

Quit smoking

Cigarette smoke harms nearly every organ of your body, and your eyes are no exception. Smoke can irritate and redden your eyes. Smoking is a risk factor for cataracts, macular degeneration, retinal vascular occlusions and more.

Eat for your eyes

Scientists believe that a lack of certain nutrients, including some vitamins, carotenoids and fats, may be why your macula and other parts of the eye may start to deteriorate with age. Upping your intake of these nutrients may help protect your eyes from age-related macular degeneration and other diseases. The best way to get these nutrients is to eat a variety of fruits and vegetables, especially those that are richly colored. The most colorful fruits and vegetables — yellow, orange, red, blue and dark green — contain nutrients that are most highly concentrated in your eyes.

Fish, which contains omega-3 fatty acids, is important to eye health and may reduce your risk of macular degeneration. Omega-3 fatty acids can also be found in lesser amounts in flaxseed, chia seeds, walnuts and canola oil.

Take care of your health

Caring for your cardiovascular health will help protect against eye disease, including retinal vessel occlusions. Avoiding diabetes will protect you against diabetic retinopathy. More than 40% of Americans with diabetes have some stage of diabetic retinopathy, a disease that damages blood vessels in the eyes. Diabetes also puts you at risk of other diseases, such as cataracts and glaucoma.

HEARING

Hearing allows you to have meaningful conversations and to experience the world around you. Problems with your hearing can chip away at your self-confidence, affect how well you communicate, and make life less enjoyable overall.

That's why protecting your hearing is such an important part of healthy aging.

Your ability to hear is orchestrated by three complex interconnected ear sections, known as the outer ear, middle ear and inner ear. The cupped shape of the outer ear gathers sound waves from the environment around you. The waves are directed into the ear canal, where they cause your eardrum to vibrate. The middle ear is an air-filled cavity behind the eardrum that houses three tiny bones called ossicles. Together, the ossicles form a bridge between the eardrum and the membrane-covered entrance to the inner ear. Each of the bones moves back and forth, much like a small lever, to increase the sound level that reaches the inner ear. The inner ear contains the most sophisticated part of the hearing mechanism: the fluid-filled, snail-shaped cochlea. The cochlea translates incoming sound waves into signals that can be understood by the brain.

Hearing loss is more common with age due to gradual degeneration of the structures of your inner ear, though a decline in hearing can occur at any age from noise exposure, trauma, genetics and illness. About 1 in 3 Americans between ages 65 and 74 has hearing loss and 1 in 2 among adults over age 75.

Age-related hearing loss

Age-related hearing loss, known as presbycusis, gradually occurs as a result of the body's natural aging process and accumulated physical and environmental factors. It's one of the most common problems affecting older adults.

There are many causes of age-related hearing loss. Most commonly, it arises from changes in the inner ear, but it can also result from changes in the middle ear, from complex changes along the nerve pathways from the ear to the brain, or in conjunction with the cumulative effects of long-term noise exposure.

Age-related hearing loss most often occurs in both ears, affecting them equally. Because the loss of hearing is gradual and subtle, you may not realize that you've lost some of your ability to hear.

Hearing changes generally first begin with difficulty detecting high-pitched sounds in both ears, followed by difficulty discerning consonants and understanding speech in noisy places, though not in quiet places. Physical changes include the ear canal getting thinner, stickier ear wax and stiffer ossicles, making it harder for the tiny bones to conduct sound.

Hearing loss and other health conditions

Preserving your hearing is important because studies have found that hearing loss may increase your risk of other health conditions, including cognitive decline, falls and depression. Individuals with mild hearing impairment are twice as likely to develop dementia compared with adults with typical hearing. The risk increases threefold if you have moderate hearing loss, and fivefold if you have severe impairment.

There are several theories regarding the hearing and dementia link. Researchers believe the connection may be due to people with hearing loss straining to decode sounds, increasing the mental effort and attention required by the brain (cognitive load).

In other words, hearing loss can make the brain work harder at the expense of other brain functions. There's also the possibility that hearing loss causes the brain to shrink more quickly. And then there's lack of social stimulation. If you can't hear very well, you may not go out as much, so the brain is less engaged and active, which is crucial to keeping intellectually stimulated.

Age-related hearing loss can also impact mental health. Losing the ability to easily communicate and understand friends and family can be isolating. Difficulty hearing can decrease the amount of enjoyment a person has in their relationships. And it can negatively impact a person's ability to stay in the workforce.

Studies suggest that having other health conditions may increase your risk of experiencing hearing loss. Cardiovascular disease can exaggerate the degree of hearing decline. Risk of hearing impairment has been found to be greater in people with hardening of the arteries (atherosclerosis) than in individuals without blood vessel abnormalities, suggesting that hearing loss could be an early sign of cardiovascular disease.

Hearing loss also is more common in individuals with diabetes, possibly due to nerve and blood vessel damage in the inner ear. People with kidney disease also appear to be at greater risk of hearing loss.

Conditions that aren't typical

For many individuals, as they get older hearing well tends to become more difficult. But not all hearing loss is simply due to age. Though fairly to somewhat common, the following conditions aren't a normal part of aging.

Conductive hearing loss

When something keeps sound waves from passing through the outer and middle ear, sound becomes muffled or faint. This is known as conductive hearing loss. Common causes of conductive hearing loss include too much earwax, a ruptured eardrum or an infection that causes fluid to build up in the middle ear. Other causes include cysts and benign tumors.

Problems with the outer ear and middle ear generally don't cause permanent damage. Conductive hearing loss can often be reversed with treatment. Sometimes, simple self-care is enough. Other times, you may need medication or surgery.

Tinnitus

Tinnitus is the name for sound in your ear that has no apparent external source. The sound is often characterized as a ringing, buzzing, whistling, chirping, hissing, humming, roaring or clicking noise.

Many people experience brief episodes of ringing or hissing in the ears after being exposed to extremely loud noise or taking certain medications. After a few hours or days, the sound usually goes away. With tinnitus, the sound is ongoing (chronic). It's estimated that up to 20 million Americans experience chronic tinnitus.

Tinnitus frequently, though not always, occurs along with hearing loss. Its impact on people's lives ranges from annoying to debilitating. Frustration with the disorder can lead to an increased risk of depression and anxiety. The good news is that tinnitus generally isn't a serious threat to your hearing or an indication of another health concern. While there's no cure for the condition, there are ways to manage it and lessen its effects. This may include using hearing aids and reviewing your medications to make sure they aren't worsening your symptoms.

Meniere's disease

This condition is characterized by spontaneous episodes of fluctuating hearing loss, tinnitus and the feeling of a plugged ear. It's often followed by a sensation of spinning or rotating (vertigo), nausea and vomiting. An attack may last from 20 minutes to several hours.

No one knows what causes Meniere's disease, but scientists link its signs and symptoms to changes in the amount of fluid in the inner ear. Too much fluid increases pressure on the membranes of the inner ear, which may distort and occasionally rupture them. This, in turn, affects hearing.

Sudden deafness

If you lose your hearing all at once or within a few days, it's considered sudden sensorineural hearing loss (SSNHL). The condition almost always affects just one ear. Many people notice a popping sound when it happens to them. They may detect hearing loss when they first wake up or try to use the affected ear. Dizziness or tinnitus may develop around the same time.

Most of the time the cause is unknown, but SSNHL may result from a viral inner ear infection, abrupt disruption of blood flow to the cochlea, a membrane tear within the cochlea or a benign tumor (acoustic neuroma). Depending on the cause, hearing loss may be permanent. If you experience sudden hearing loss, seek medical attention right away.

What you can do

Because hearing changes are subtle, it's important to have your ears checked regularly, even though hearing tests generally aren't a standard part of medical exams. If you're concerned about hearing loss or you've been in a situation that increases your risk of hearing loss, you can ask for a hearing exam. In addition, there are other steps that you can take:

Be careful with listening devices

Many people use personal devices such as headphones or earbuds to listen to music or other media. Unfortunately, some users listen for too long at too high a volume. This can cause noise-induced hearing loss, which you may overlook until your hearing has been significantly damaged. When using personal listening devices, keep the volume at a level where you can still carry on a conversation. An indication the volume may be too loud is that after listening, sounds are muffled or your ears are ringing.

Wear hearing protection

Loud noises from recreational, industrial and military activities can increase risk of hearing loss. In these settings, plastic earplugs or glycerin-filled earmuffs can help protect your ears from damaging noise. Activities such as mowing the lawn, riding a snowmobile, using power tools, hunting or attending rock concerts can damage your hearing over time. Consider using special earmuffs at high-intensity venues such as the gun range.

Protect your blood vessels

Good cardiovascular health ensures that the small blood vessels in your ear receive enough oxygenated blood to help protect against damage to the ear's tiny structures, which can result in hearing loss. Diabetes can damage blood vessels and nerves in the ear; according to some estimates, hearing loss is twice as common in people who have diabetes as in people who don't.

Take care of your bones

Strong bones are critical to hearing because your inner ear is housed in the temporal bone. Bone loss in the temporal bone may lead to inner ear damage, resulting in hearing loss. Bone loss can affect the tiny bones within your inner ear (ossicles), which help transport sound waves to your brain. Reduced bone density may alter the chemical processes required for your inner ear to function properly.

Exercise

Inactivity is linked to hearing loss in older adults. Fortunately, the reverse is also true. Individuals who are physically active are less likely to experience hearing loss. Exercise gets your heart pumping and oxygen flowing. It's one of the best ways to keep the blood vessels in your ears healthy. Aim for at least 30 minutes of activity each day. Even short bouts of activity offer benefits.

Eat healthy

A healthy diet can protect against hearing loss in many ways. For one, it helps lower blood pressure and cholesterol, which keeps blood flowing smoothly through your blood vessels. That ensures blood flows well to your inner ear. Good nutrition also keeps your brain functioning well and protects the nerve pathways between your ears and your brain. A low-calorie diet that limits salt, saturated fat and sugar and emphasizes fruits and vegetables can help reduce your risk of hearing loss.

SMELL

Your nose is a gateway to your respiratory system, allowing air to travel to your lungs. It's also responsible for your sense of smell and to a large degree your sense of taste, because your ability to taste depends on your sense of smell.

Smell begins at the top of your nasal cavity, where small nerve fibers pierce the interface between your brain and your nose. These fibers react with molecules in the air, generating a signal to a larger nerve associated with smell, which delivers the signal of smell to your brain.

In addition to affecting how you taste and appreciate food, your sense of smell helps you enjoy a walk in the woods, a bouquet of spring flowers or your reliable morning coffee. Smells also help us recall a memory, such as a mother's perfume or a favorite bakery. And they keep us safe, warning us of dangers such as smoke, gas or spoiled food.

As you get older, especially once you reach your 70s, you may notice a decline in your smell acuity. This happens because of a decrease in nerve fibers within structures in your nose (olfactory bulbs) involved in the sense of smell. As a result, smells don't register as strongly, and it becomes a bit more challenging to differentiate between different smells.

Loss of smell can have a significant impact on your quality of life. It can lead to decreased appetite and poor nutrition. It can sometimes contribute to depression. Loss of smell might also tempt you to use excess salt or sugar on your food to enhance the taste.

Conditions that aren't typical

While a decrease in smell acuity is common with age, loss of smell can occur for other reasons. If you lose your sense of smell suddenly or loss of smell is accompanied by other symptoms, talk to your health care provider to see if there's an underlying medical condition involved. Sometimes, loss of smell may be a sign of a more serious disorder, such as mild cognitive impairment, Alzheimer's disease or Parkinson's disease.

Most conditions that produce a loss of smell, such as a cold, influenza or allergies, are temporary or can be treated. Other conditions that can affect your sense of smell include:

- **COVID-19.** Infection with the virus known as severe acute respiratory syndrome coronavirus 2 (SARS-CoV-2) can cause some people to lose their sense of smell. Most people regain their ability to smell after a few days when their symptoms improve.
- **Polyps.** These pearl-like lumps caused by swelling of the nasal membranes

can block nasal passages, affecting your ability to smell. Loss of the sense of smell may also occur if the olfactory area or its nerve fibers are damaged.

- **Medications.** Some medications can reduce your smell acuity, including over-the-counter nasal sprays that contain zinc.

What you can do

There are a few things that you can do to help preserve your sense of smell. They include exercising, avoiding excessive use of alcohol and tobacco products, and not using cleaning products with strong fumes.

Smell rehabilitation, also called olfactory therapy, is sometimes used to help regain your sense of smell or help strengthen it. Therapists work with scented oils to rewire the brain's ability to process and differentiate odors.

If you've lost your sense of smell and worry about safety issues such as being able to detect gas or something burning or protecting yourself from eating rotting food, take precautions. Make sure your home has working smoke and carbon monoxide detectors. Label food so that you know when it's no longer safe and should be thrown out.

TASTE

Your sense of taste and sense of smell are intricately connected. When you eat something, you experience its flavor based on five basic tastes — sweet, salty, bitter, sour and savory — as well as the sensations of heat and coolness. A food's flavor is also influenced by how it smells.

Similar to what happens with your sense of smell, taste acuity and taste discrimination change as you get older. Small taste buds inside your mouth — which live on your tongue, throat and the roof of the mouth — gradually lose their sensitivity. As a result, it becomes more difficult to discriminate between flavors or the gradation of flavor. In addition, a decline in the production of saliva that comes with age causes your mouth to feel drier and affects your ability to taste and decipher flavors.

The biggest risk with a reduction in taste is its impact on nutrition. If you can't taste your food, then it's not as pleasurable to eat and it becomes harder to get the calories, protein, carbohydrates, vitamins and minerals that you need for good health.

Another risk to your health is that to make up for loss of flavor, you may add more salt, fat or sugar to your foods.

Changes that aren't typical

While a decrease in taste acuity is common with age, loss of taste can occur for other reasons. If you lose your sense of taste suddenly or the loss is accompanied by other symptoms, talk to your health care provider to see if an underlying medical condition may be involved.

Most conditions that produce a loss of taste are temporary or can be treated. They include certain medications, gum disease or denture issues. A change in taste may also result from:

- **COVID-19.** Loss of taste can be a symptom of the virus that causes COVID-19. Most people regain their sense of taste after other symptoms associated with the illness have gone away. If your ability to taste doesn't return, seek medical care.
- **Salivary gland disorders.** When your mouth doesn't make enough saliva, it becomes more difficult to distinguish flavors, and food tends to lose its flavor.
- **Cancer treatment.** People receiving chemotherapy or other drug treatments for cancer often comment that food tastes "off." Some people complain that their food tastes metallic, which can affect their desire to eat. Once treatment is complete, sense of taste usually returns to normal.

What you can do

There are many ways to make eating enjoyable and your food flavorful even when your sense of taste is altered.

Keep your mouth moist

Drink plenty of water and suck on lozenges that help produce saliva. You also can purchase over-the-counter products intended to increase saliva production. Generally, the more saliva you have, the better your food will taste.

Try a saline rinse

If your loss of taste is related to a reduction in your sense of smell due to allergies or a cold, try an over-the-counter nasal saline solution. These products rinse your nasal passages and sinuses and can help improve your smell, thereby improving your sense of taste.

Experiment with colors and spices

If you're having trouble smelling and tasting your food, adding color and texture to make your food more interesting may help. For example, try eating brightly colored vegetables and fruits.

Also, use herbs and spices such as sage, thyme, rosemary, oregano, cinnamon and nutmeg to add flavor to your meals. To put some zing in your foods, add mustard, onions, garlic, ginger, spices or lemon or lime juice. These flavor enhancers are better than salt, especially if you have high blood pressure.

TOUCH

Your skin is an amazing organ covering the surface of your body. It contains millions of tiny sensors that detect feeling in many different forms. Sensations gathered from your skin's receptors are transmitted via your nerves to your brain, where they're interpreted.

Our sense of touch provides our brain a wealth of information about our natural environment. More importantly, it allows us to experience many different feelings — the joy and comfort in a hug from a loved one, the warmth and gentleness of a soft sweater, the calm and relaxation of a gentle breeze. All of these pleasurable feelings are important to healthy aging.

Our sense of touch also helps protect us from injury. Skin sensors warn us to let go of a hot object, be careful with objects that feel sharp or remove ourselves from circumstances that cause pain.

The same age-related changes that impact your senses of smell and taste also affect your sense of touch. Touch acuity weakens or changes with time. Often times, changes affecting touch are associated with decreased blood flow to the body's nerve endings or to the brain.

Conditions that aren't typical

Sometimes alterations to the body's sense of touch go beyond normal aging and can be a warning of a more serious health concern. Malnutrition, brain surgery or injury and nerve damage from long-term (chronic) diseases such as diabetes can also alter or diminish your sensation of touch.

Peripheral neuropathy results from damage to the nerves located outside your brain and spinal cord (peripheral nerves). When the peripheral nerves are injured, you may experience numbness, pain and weakness, usually in the hands and feet.

A common cause of peripheral neuropathy is diabetes. In some situations, the condition may be associated with changes in digestion, urination and circulation. It may result from traumatic injuries, infections, metabolic problems, inherited diseases and exposure to toxins.

What you can do

To help preserve your sense of touch and reduce your risk of neuropathy, it's important to keep your nerves healthy. To help maintain touch acuity:

Get enough B-12

Make sure to include plenty of fruits, vegetables, whole grains and lean protein in your diet. These foods help protect against nerve damage by making sure you get adequate vitamin B-12. Vitamin B-12 helps produce a substance called myelin, a protective coating that shields the nerves and helps them transmit sensations. Other foods that contain vitamin B-12 include fish, eggs, low-fat dairy items and fortified cereals.

Protect your nerves

Moderate aerobic exercise helps preserve peripheral nerve function. Try to get at least 30 to 60 minutes of exercise three times a week.

At the same time, avoid circumstances that can damage your nerves. These include use of repetitive motions, cramped positions that put pressure on your nerves, exposure to toxic chemicals, smoking and excessive alcohol. If you have diabetes, talk to your health care provider about ways to improve your blood sugar control.

As your senses change over time, it's important to preserve those faculties and sensations that are still functioning well. Even a few small steps can help you continue to enjoy the world around you.

WHAT DO YOU THINK?

As you reflect on what you just read and contemplate your future health, ask yourself these questions.

- *How do I feel about my current sensory health?*
- *What am I doing now that I feel good about?*
- *What are some aspects of my sensory health I'd like to improve?*
- *What changes can I make that I'm most likely to stick with?*

Your heart and lungs

The heart is the body's most powerful organ — each day beating about 100,000 times and pumping approximately 80 gallons of blood an hour to bring oxygen and nutrients to all tissues of the body. Given the complex and essential function of this organ, it's not surprising that even moderate impairments in heart function can have significant consequences on overall health.

Diseases of the heart and blood vessels aren't a given as you get older. However, cardiovascular disease poses the greatest threat to longevity. It's the No. 1 cause of death in both men and women. Approximately 700,000 Americans die each year from cardiovascular disease.

It's estimated that at least 80% of all cardiovascular disease is preventable through diet, exercise and quitting smoking. As with many aspects of health, prevention begins in young adulthood.

YOUR HEART

The flow of blood through your heart and circulatory system is an intricate process. With age, things can change inside and outside the heart, leading to different forms of disease. If blood flow is interrupted, problems can develop quickly and cascade throughout the rest of your body. Many forms of cardiovascular disease can lead to heart failure, meaning that your heart can't pump enough blood to meet your body's needs.

Fortunately, most cardiovascular diseases progress slowly over many years, so even small steps toward a healthier lifestyle early in life can accumulate to result in substantially better heart health — or completely prevent many cardiovascular diseases — with age. Because several of the strongest risk factors for cardiovascular disease are things you can change, you have far more control over the health of your heart and blood vessels than you may realize.

Heart function

Your heart is a muscular organ about the size of your fist. It has four separate chambers and four valves that function as one-way doors. It also has its own electrical system that triggers each heartbeat.

Your heart works closely with your lungs. The right side of your heart is responsible for collecting oxygen-depleted blood and waste from your body, such as carbon dioxide, which is produced by your tissues, and sending it to your lungs. The left side of your heart receives oxygen-rich blood from your lungs and pumps it out to fuel your body's cells. Blood pumped from the heart travels to the rest of the body by way of your arteries and travels back to your heart and lungs by way of your veins. The heart's blood supply comes from arteries that wrap around it, known as the coronary arteries.

Your heart also works hand in hand with your brain. The brain can signal the heart to speed up or slow down and can regulate pressure within your circulatory system by contracting or relaxing your blood vessels. The pressure resulting from blood moving through your veins and arteries is known as your blood pressure.

With age, changes commonly occur within the heart and circulatory system, causing the system to become less efficient. If the changes are significant, they can lead to disease and disability.

Common age-related changes

Aging naturally causes several changes in your heart and blood vessels. In some individuals these changes begin sooner than in others.

Artery stiffening

The most common change with age is stiffening of your artery walls. Healthy arteries are flexible and elastic, but over time walls in the arteries can harden, causing them to lose their elasticity. This makes your heart work harder to pump blood through the arteries and causes your blood pressure to rise as blood moves through the arteries. The medical term for thickening and hardening of your artery walls is arteriosclerosis.

Artery narrowing

Over time, fat and other substances can accumulate in the arteries, forming deposits called plaques. As plaques form, the arteries can narrow. The medical term for this condition is atherosclerosis.

Atherosclerosis is thought to start from injury or damage to an artery's inner layer, a thin lining of cells inside your blood vessels called the endothelium. The damage may result from many causes, including high cholesterol levels, tobacco use, high blood pressure, diabetes and inflammation.

Increased cholesterol

Cholesterol is a waxy, fatlike substance in your blood. Too much cholesterol can lead to an increase in the formation of plaques. Cholesterol levels tend to increase from ages 16 to 60, and some people develop elevated cholesterol levels at a young age. Plaques and fatty streaks have been identified in people in their 20s. While some research suggests that after age 60 cholesterol levels may decline in some individuals, in women they generally increase after menopause. Maintaining healthy blood cholesterol is one of the best ways to prevent heart disease.

Heart valve thickening and weakening

The heart's valves are like one-way shutters that open and close to control the pace of blood flow through the heart's four chambers. Your heart valves open and shut tens of thousands of times a day. With age, the valves can thicken and stiffen, limiting the flow of blood out of your heart (valve stenosis). The heart's valves also may deteriorate and not close properly, causing blood to leak back into the chamber instead of being expelled (valve regurgitation). When heart valve stenosis or regurgitation becomes severe, fluid can build up in the lungs, legs, feet and abdomen.

Heart rhythm changes

The heart has a natural pacemaker system that controls how fast it beats. Over time, fibrous tissue and fat deposits may form in the pathways of this electrical system, and the heart's natural pacemaker, called the sinus node, may lose some of its cells. These changes may result in a slower or irregular heart rate. Abnormal heart rhythms (arrhythmias) also become more common with age. Many people experience occasional fluttering of the heart, especially during stressful times or when exercising. This is because parts of the heart tissue have the ability to become excited or irritated. Arrhythmias can happen for a number of reasons and generally aren't cause for alarm. Problems can occur, however, when an abnormal rhythm persists for a longer period of time or makes you feel unwell.

Reduced blood pressure control

Receptors within some of your blood vessels (baroreceptors) monitor your blood pressure and make changes to

ABNORMAL RESPONSE TO HEALING

An interesting fact about the heart is that it doesn't respond like other parts of your body to injury and healing. When you cut your hand, for instance, your body activates specific molecular pathways that trigger your cells to build more fibrous tissue and heal the cut, which can often result in the formation of a scar. Your body recruits immune cells to create a controlled inflammatory response and fight off infection.

Your body applies the same approach to healing in the cardiovascular system that it does to other injured tissues in your body. But these healing mechanisms don't always result in a beneficial outcome when activated in cardiovascular tissues. They produce fibrous tissue or calcifications where you don't want them, which can cause stiffening of your heart muscle and coronary arteries. This is part of the reason why injury to heart tissues can have a cascading effect.

help maintain a fairly constant blood pressure, especially when you change positions or perform certain activities. Baroreceptors generally become less sensitive with age, in part because your blood vessels become stiffer. This is why your blood pressure may drop and you may become a bit dizzy when moving from a sitting to a standing position too quickly, what's known as orthostatic hypotension. The drop in blood pressure causes less blood flow to the brain, triggering a brief episode of dizziness.

Decreased blood volume

Your total amount of blood supply changes slightly with age. Normal aging causes a reduction in total body water. As a result, there's less fluid in the bloodstream, causing a small decrease in blood volume.

Keep in mind that just because changes to your heart and circulatory system with age are common, it doesn't mean they're guaranteed. Some aspects of heart and blood vessel aging can be slowed or reversed with healthy lifestyle choices, such as exercise, a healthy diet, not smoking, and controlling stress. Research indicates that improvements in heart and blood vessel function can occur rapidly with regular exercise, so it's never too late to adopt a healthier lifestyle.

CONDITIONS THAT AREN'T TYPICAL

Minor changes to your heart and blood vessels generally aren't a problem. But more severe changes can lead to development of significant cardiovascular disease that impacts your quality of life. And, not surprisingly, changes beget changes — development of one condition often leads to another.

Following are the most common heart-related conditions and factors that increase your risk. You aren't destined to develop these diseases as you age, but your chances increase the older you get, especially if you have several risk factors.

Coronary artery disease

The coronary arteries are those that encircle and supply blood to your heart. When these arteries become damaged or blocked, either partially or completely, the condition is known as coronary artery disease.

Coronary artery disease typically develops over many years. It starts with small changes in the inner lining of a coronary artery that injure or damage cells so that the cells stop working properly. Factors that often contribute to this damage include smoking, high

WARNINGS OF A HEART ATTACK

Not all people who have a heart attack experience the same signs and symptoms or experience them to the same degree. In addition, heart attack symptoms in women, older adults and individuals with diabetes tend to be less pronounced. Some people have no symptoms at all. Still, there often are warnings that a heart attack may be occurring:

- Pressure, fullness or a squeezing pain in the center of your chest that lasts more than a few minutes.
- Pain that extends to your shoulder, arm, back or even to your teeth and jaw.
- Increasing episodes of chest pain.
- Prolonged pain in the upper abdomen.
- Shortness of breath during exercise or at rest.
- Unusual feeling of fatigue during normal activities.
- Sweating.
- Lightheadedness or fainting.
- Nausea and vomiting.

Many people who experience a heart attack have mild warning signs and symptoms for hours, days or weeks in advance.

Just like when your other muscles experience a burning sensation when they don't get enough blood during intense exercise (because of a buildup of substances called metabolites), the heart muscle accumulates metabolites and activates similar sensing pathways when it doesn't get enough blood. In the heart, however, this feels like a sensation of deep pressure or pain, and the earliest predictor of an attack may be recurrent chest pressure or pain triggered by exertion and relieved by rest, a condition called angina.

blood pressure, high cholesterol, diabetes, infections and the aging process.

As with any type of injury, cell damage often triggers inflammation. Deposits that contain fat and cholesterol (plaques) tend to accumulate at the site of the injury. As plaques form, artery walls thicken. Eventually, plaque accumulation reaches the point that the blood vessel becomes narrowed and blood flow is reduced.

Your heart may get enough blood to fuel normal activities of daily living, such as sitting or standing at work or doing daily chores around your house. But when the heart has to work harder, such as during exercise, it needs more blood, and the narrowed and thickened arteries can't meet the demand. Reduced blood flow to your heart can cause chest pain (angina). You may also experience shortness of breath.

Occasionally, plaques in an artery may crack or rupture. In response, blood particles clump together at the site to repair the crack. The particles form a blood clot that can completely block the artery and cut off the blood supply, leading to a heart attack. Some people aren't aware that they have coronary artery disease until they've had a heart attack.

Are you at risk?

Several factors place you at added risk of coronary artery disease. Some you can control, and others you can't.

Uncontrollable risk factors for coronary artery disease include:
- **Sex.** Men are generally at greater risk of heart disease than women. However, after menopause, the risk of heart disease increases in women. Despite this difference, cardiovascular disease is the leading cause of death in both men and women.
- **Heredity.** If your siblings, parents or grandparents had coronary artery disease, you may be at risk, too. Your family may have a genetic condition contributing to higher blood cholesterol levels or high blood pressure. Knowing your family history is important when planning the best approaches to preventing cardiovascular disease.
- **Race.** Black people and those of Latino, Native American and Native Hawaiian races generally have a higher risk of heart disease and high blood pressure than do white people.
- **Age.** Your risk of developing significant coronary artery disease increases with age.

Controllable risk factors for coronary artery disease include:

- **Smoking.** Exposure to cigarette smoke and other factors greatly increase your risk of coronary artery disease by damaging blood vessels and promoting inflammation.
- **High blood pressure.** Over time, high blood pressure can damage the coronary arteries by accelerating plaque formation and artery wall stiffening.
- **High blood cholesterol.** Risk of coronary artery disease increases as your blood cholesterol level rises, especially if the level of low-density lipoprotein (LDL, or "bad") cholesterol is high.
- **Diabetes.** Individuals with diabetes have an increased risk of coronary artery disease, and the risk is higher if their blood sugar level isn't well controlled.
- **Obesity.** Excess weight increases strain on your heart, raises your blood pressure, increases your blood cholesterol levels, and increases your risk of diabetes.
- **An unhealthy diet.** Eating foods containing a lot of saturated fat, trans fat, salt and sugar can increase your disease risk.
- **Inactivity.** The less physically active you are, the greater your risk of coronary artery disease.
- **Stress and anger.** Strong emotions can increase your risk. This is especially true if they trigger other risk factors, such as overeating or smoking.
- **Excessive alcohol consumption.** Drinking too much alcohol can lead to several factors that increase the risk of coronary artery disease, including increased blood pressure, increased blood triglycerides, development of inflammation and formation of blood clots.

Risk factors may feed one another. For example, obesity commonly leads to diabetes and high blood pressure. Even a small increase in one factor becomes more critical when combined with others.

High blood pressure

When your heart pumps, it generates pressure in your blood vessels to move blood throughout your body. Pressure created by this pumping action is your blood pressure. When the force of blood against your artery wall is high for a long time, the cells in the blood vessel wall try to adapt to this stress.

One way blood vessels adapt to high blood pressure is by becoming thicker and less elastic. While this prevents them from bulging out or rupturing, it can decrease the flow of blood and oxygen to your heart and can make blood pressure go even higher. If the arteries that supply blood and oxygen to your brain become damaged and clogged or if blood pressure becomes too high, a stroke can result. High blood pressure (hypertension) can lead to several other conditions throughout your body.

Blood pressure is measured using two numbers. The first (top) number, called systolic blood pressure, measures the pressure in your arteries when your heart beats. The second number (bottom), called diastolic blood pressure, measures the pressure in your arteries when your heart rests between beats.

Your blood pressure is considered normal when your systolic pressure is 120 millimeters of mercury (mm Hg) or less and your diastolic pressure is at or below 80 mm Hg.

BLOOD PRESSURE CLASSIFICATIONS

The American College of Cardiology and the American Heart Association divide blood pressure into four general categories.

Normal blood pressure. Blood pressure is 120/80 millimeters of mercury (mm Hg) or lower.

Elevated blood pressure. The top number ranges from 120 to 129 mm Hg and the bottom number is below 80 mm Hg.

Stage 1 hypertension. The top number ranges from 130 to 139 mm Hg or the bottom number is between 80 and 89 mm Hg.

Stage 2 hypertension. The top number is 140 mm Hg or higher or the bottom number is 90 mm Hg or higher.

120/80

↓

140/90

Are you at risk?

Several factors place you at added risk of high blood pressure. Again, some you can control, and others you can't. Uncontrollable risk factors include:

- **Age.** Risk of high blood pressure increases with age. Until about age 64, high blood pressure is more common in men. Women are more likely to develop high blood pressure after age 65.
- **Race.** High blood pressure is particularly common in Black individuals, and it often develops at an earlier age in this group than in other races.
- **Family history.** You're more likely to develop high blood pressure if you have a parent or sibling with the condition.

Controllable risk factors for coronary artery disease include:

- **Obesity or being overweight.** Excess weight triggers changes that can affect your blood vessels and kidneys. These changes often increase blood pressure.
- **Inactivity.** Too little physical activity can cause weight gain. Increased weight raises the risk of high blood pressure. People who are inactive also tend to have increased heart rates.
- **Tobacco use or vaping.** Smoking, chewing tobacco or vaping immediately raises blood pressure for a short while. Smoking injures blood vessel walls, speeds up the process of hardening the arteries and contributes to long-term high blood pressure that is difficult to treat or reverse.
- **Too much salt.** Excess salt (sodium) can cause your body to retain fluid. This increases blood pressure.
- **Low electrolyte levels.** Potassium and magnesium help balance the amount of salt in the body's cells. A proper balance of potassium is important for good heart health. Low potassium levels may be due to a lack of potassium in the diet or certain health conditions, including dehydration.
- **Too much alcohol.** Excess alcohol consumption has been linked to increased blood pressure.
- **Stress.** High levels of stress can lead to a temporary increase in blood pressure. Stress-related habits such as overeating, using tobacco or drinking alcohol can result in further increases.

Arrhythmias

Heart rhythm problems, called arrhythmias, often are harmless. But they can be an indication of a more serious heart condition. Arrhythmias result from abnormalities in the pathway that the heart's electrical signals travel in order to make your heart beat. Faulty signaling can cause the heart to beat too fast (tachycardia), too slow (bradycardia) or irregularly.

Sometimes arrhythmias are hereditary. Other times they may stem from underlying heart disease that affects the structure of the heart or causes scarring in the heart muscle. Other problems such as high blood pressure, diabetes, a thyroid disorder or a sleep disorder can disturb the heart's rhythm. Beverages or medications that stimulate the heart also may trigger abnormal heart rhythms.

Are you at risk?

Factors that increase risk of a heart arrhythmia include:

- **High blood pressure.** This can cause the walls of the lower-left heart chamber (left ventricle) to stiffen and thicken, which can change how electrical signals travel through the heart.
- **Other heart conditions.** Narrowed arteries within the heart can reduce blood flow to parts of the heart and speed up or slow down the heart's normal rhythm. Heart valve disorders can also affect the heart's normal rhythm.
- **Congenital heart disease.** Being born with a heart condition may affect the heart's rhythm and increase your lifetime risk for arrhythmias.
- **Thyroid disease.** Having an overactive or underactive thyroid gland can raise the risk of experiencing irregular heartbeats.
- **Obstructive sleep apnea.** This causes pauses in breathing during sleep, which can lead to slow and irregular heartbeats. Sleep apnea also increases your risk for high blood pressure during the day.
- **Electrolyte imbalance.** Substances in blood called electrolytes — such as potassium, sodium, calcium and magnesium — help trigger and send electrical impulses in the heart. An imbalance in electrolytes — for example, being too high or too low — can interfere with heart signaling and lead to irregular heartbeats.
- **Certain drugs and supplements.** Some prescription medications and certain cough and cold medications bought without a prescription can cause arrhythmias.
- **Caffeine, nicotine or illegal drug use.** Caffeine, nicotine and other stimulants can cause your heart to beat faster and may lead to the development of more serious arrhythmias. Illegal drugs, such as amphetamines and cocaine, can greatly affect the heart and lead to many types of arrhythmias or sudden death.

Heart valve disorders

Four valves keep blood flowing through the chambers of the heart. They consist of strong, thin flaps of tissue (leaflets) that open and close with each heartbeat. The valves allow blood to flow in one direction throughout the heart.

With a heart valve disorder, one of the valves fails to open or close properly, generally due to tissue weakening, stiffening or deterioration over time. This can result in two problems: narrowing of the valve opening (stenosis) and leakage of blood back through the valve opening (regurgitation).

Heart valve disorders can develop for a variety of reasons. They include:

- **Calcium buildup.** Calcium is a mineral present in all of your cells and in your bloodstream. As you age, however, increases in blood pressure, high cholesterol or other risk factors can result in the deposition of calcium on the heart valve that lets blood flow out of the heart (aortic valve). These deposits thicken and stiffen the valve leaflets, narrowing the valve's opening and limiting the flow of blood out of the heart. This is called aortic valve stenosis.
- **Wear and tear.** Your valves open and shut thousands of times each day, and over time they may weaken or deteriorate. When they don't close tightly and blood flows in the wrong direction, it's called valvular regurgitation.
- **Infection.** Rheumatic fever, a complication of untreated strep throat infections, can damage the heart's valves. Infection inside the heart (endocarditis) also can lead to heart valve disease.
- **Birth defect.** Some people are born with a heart valve defect in which there is an abnormal number of heart valves or the valves don't function properly.

Are you at risk?

Factors that can put you at increased risk of a heart valve disorder include:

- **Age.** Older age can be a risk factor, especially if your lifestyle habits also raise your risk. Notably, increasing age is the strongest risk factor for development of aortic valve stenosis.
- **Family history.** Some valve disorders run in families. Given some of the shared risk factors between coronary artery disease and heart valve disease, a family history of early coronary artery disease also may increase your risk of developing heart valve disease.
- **Lifestyle habits.** Factors that can increase your risk for other types of

heart disease, such as an unhealthy diet, smoking and obesity, may put you at risk for development or accelerated progression of heart valve diseases.

- **Other conditions.** High blood pressure, diabetes, autoimmune disorders such as lupus and other heart conditions can increase your risk of heart valve disease.
- **Radiation treatment.** Radiation therapy to the chest, a common treatment for some cancers, may lead to thickening and narrowing of the heart valves.

EARLY INTERVENTION

The most crucial step in preventing cardiovascular disease is addressing risk factors early. No matter your background or medical history, it's always a good idea to talk to your primary care provider about your individual risk of heart disease and a heart-healthy lifestyle.

Age-related changes in blood cholesterol, blood pressure and artery wall stiffening naturally increase your risk of cardiovascular disease. If you view these small changes as occasional snow flurries, you may think that you don't need to worry about each individual snowflake. The challenge, however, is that flurries can accumulate and form

into a snowball that may start rolling downhill. The goal is to minimize snowball formation and, if a snowball has already formed, keep it from growing and gaining momentum as it continues on a downhill trajectory.

If you have moderately increased blood cholesterol levels, elevated blood pressure or prediabetes, early management and intervention should be a priority. Cardiovascular disease becomes more difficult to treat in its more advanced stages, and late stages of the disease may require surgery. Also, the longer these conditions progress unchecked, the greater your risk of a heart attack or stroke that can dramatically affect your independence and reduce your quality of life.

The best strategies for preventing and managing heart disease are adopting heart-healthy lifestyle habits, seeing your health care provider on a regular basis and getting recommended screenings (see pages 278-279).

Additional heart-health risks

As part of your screening, your provider may inquire about other circumstances known to influence heart health. Most factors that place people at increased risk of cardiovascular disease come as no surprise — tobacco use, too much alcohol, too little exercise, an unhealthy diet and poor sleep, which commonly occurs with sleep apnea.

There are additional risks to your heart and circulatory system that you may not be aware of, such as chronic stress, working night shifts and environmental pollutants. These can also increase risk of a heart attack or stroke.

Chronic stress

Persistent or severe stress can occur for many reasons. Chronic stress is associated

TRACKING YOUR HEART HEALTH

These are the tests most often used to monitor the health of your heart and circulatory system and how often you should have them.

Test	How often?
Blood pressure measurement	Every health care visit. Once a year if your blood pressure is lower than 120/80 mm Hg. More frequently if it's higher.
Blood cholesterol test (fasting lipoprotein profile)	Every 4 to 6 years if you're at normal risk of cardiovascular disease. More often if you have an elevated risk of heart disease and stroke.
Blood sugar (glucose) test	Every 3 years if the results are normal. More frequently if you have prediabetes or diabetes.
Weight/body mass index (BMI)	Every health care visit. Once a year if your weight is healthy. More often if your BMI indicates you're overweight or obese.
Smoking, physical activity and dietary assessment	Yearly.

with a complex physiologic response that may lead to several physical changes, including an increased heart rate and increases in blood pressure. Persistent stress may also trigger chronic inflammation within your heart and arteries.

Stress also affects cardiovascular health in indirect ways. When you're worried or anxious, you may sleep poorly, overeat, eat unhealthy foods, consume more alcohol and use tobacco — all known risk factors for heart disease.

Night-shift work

Research involving individuals who work night shifts indicate a slight to moderate increased risk of coronary artery disease compared to those who don't work night shifts. Studies also suggest the risk of disease increases with the more nights worked and is greater among people who work rotating night shifts — that is, who switch back and forth between day and night work.

Disruption to the body's biological (circadian) rhythms, sleep issues and abnormal eating patterns associated with shift work are believed to be the main culprits for poorer heart health. Some studies also suggest that individuals who work night shifts tend to weigh

more than those who work traditional day shifts. And there's some indication that people who work night shifts are less socially active, which can increase stress and feelings of isolation as a result of fewer social connections.

Environmental pollutants

Tiny pollution particles in the air can affect your lung function, which can have an indirect effect on your heart. Pollution can come from traffic, factories, power generation, wildfires or even cooking with a woodstove. One of the most common indoor sources of pollution is smoking — a danger to the person smoking and to those nearby. Being aware of your exposure to environmental pollutants and doing your best to avoid them are important to your long-term cardiovascular health.

RESPONDING TO YOUR RISKS

Getting a handle on your risk factors for cardiovascular disease can be a game changer. During the last 40 years, deaths from heart disease have fallen significantly. This isn't only because people were able to identify their risks earlier and implement effective lifestyle changes but also because the tools doctors have to treat risk factors have increased dramatically during this time.

Plus, many of the steps you can take to reduce your cardiovascular risks can also boost your overall health, longevity and quality of life. For example, caring for your heart can reduce your risk for many other diseases, including cancer, diabetes, kidney disease and blindness.

The following steps can help prevent cardiovascular disease and keep your heart and circulatory system healthy as you age. If you have heart disease, these steps can often prevent your condition from worsening. You can learn more about healthy lifestyle changes and how to incorporate them into your daily routine in Part 2 of this book.

Don't smoke, and avoid secondhand smoke

Tobacco has a powerful effect on your cardiovascular system. Smoking accelerates the development of atherosclerosis and narrows your heart's blood vessels, raises blood pressure and increases your risk of blood clots. Nicotine constricts your blood vessels and forces your heart to work harder, and carbon monoxide inhaled from burning cigarettes reduces oxygen in your blood and damages the lining of your blood vessels. Being exposed to secondhand smoke can produce similar effects.

Using smokeless tobacco, or vaping, results in the same rapid delivery of nicotine throughout the body, increasing your risk of high blood pressure, blood clots and cancer. Despite what you may have heard or read, vaping isn't a safe alternative to cigarette smoking.

Quitting tobacco brings immediate benefits to your overall health, and there are medications and programs available to help you quit. If you've tried to quit before and weren't successful, don't be afraid to try again. Talk to your health care provider about options for stopping tobacco use.

Keep moving

Science and the way our bodies work tell us that we need two types of physical activity to optimize our heart health. We need to be physically active, and we need to be physically fit.

A sedentary lifestyle — spending too much time seated at a desk, in a car or in front of the television — increases your risk of death from heart disease. And between work and leisure, most people spend too much time sitting.

When it comes to your heart health, and your health in general (including your mental health), you need to do two things each day: First, keep on your feet, when possible, to avoid sitting too much. Second, engage in structured exercise.

Exercise involves performing an activity that increases your heart rate, causing you to breathe heavily and perspire. Vigorous activity leads to physical fitness. Fitness helps prevent cardiovascular disease by helping you to achieve and maintain a healthy weight, as well as control diabetes, cholesterol and your blood pressure.

As a general rule, aim for a minimum of 30 minutes of moderate exercise every day — that's less than 3% of the 16 hours most individuals are awake. More time is even better!

Start small, set achievable short-term goals and celebrate those goals when you reach them. Over time, you'll feel better, reduce your cardiovascular risk and improve your quality of life. It's important to include both aerobic activity and strength-training exercises in your exercise routine, since strength training can prevent losses in muscle mass that normally occur as you age and help you maintain a good quality of life in the future.

Eat for your heart

Too much saturated fat and cholesterol in your diet can narrow the arteries leading to your heart. Excess salt can raise your blood pressure. Oftentimes high levels of salt and saturated fats can be hidden in highly processed foods, so checking nutrition labels is a great first step toward making healthier food choices.

Shifting to a more plant-based diet composed of vegetables, fruits, whole grains, beans, nuts, unsaturated fats and lean sources of protein, such as fish, has been shown to be good for heart health and significantly reduce the risk of atherosclerosis (and in some instances, even reverse it). This type of diet can also lower blood pressure, reduce cholesterol levels and reduce your risk of coronary artery disease.

Vegetables and fruits are important because they contain antioxidants, vitamins and minerals that reduce inflammation and help prevent wear and tear on your heart muscle, coronary arteries and other blood vessels.

Whole grains, which include foods such as brown rice, quinoa, wild rice, whole-grain breakfast cereals, farro and oatmeal, help decrease LDL cholesterol in the blood. A recent meta-analysis found that people who ate the largest amounts of whole grains were 13% less likely to die of cardiovascular causes than people who ate the smallest amounts.

Fish is good for your heart and arteries because it contains omega-3 fatty acids, which help improve blood cholesterol

levels and prevent blood clots. Monounsaturated fats, such as those found in olive oil and nuts, provide the same cardiovascular health benefits as omega-3s.

Avocados, which contain unsaturated fat, also are heart-friendly. A large study published in the *Journal of the American Heart Association* found that people who ate at least two servings of avocados a week saw a 16% decrease in their risk of stroke, heart attack and death from stroke or heart attack compared with those who rarely or never ate avocados. Keep in mind, however, that avocados are higher in calories due to their higher fat content.

Maintain a healthy weight

Achieving and maintaining a healthy weight (see Chapter 9) is one of the best things you can do for your heart. Weight gain is linked to increased blood cholesterol, high blood pressure and diabetes, which can lead to coronary artery disease.

Researchers now know that excess fat is a major driver of systemic inflammation and can cause other chemical changes in blood that affect the heart and blood vessels. If you're overweight, shedding a

IT'S NEVER TOO LATE

When it comes to caring for your heart, keep in mind that not all change is permanent. Even if you've been diagnosed with heart disease, you can take steps to preserve your remaining heart function — and maybe even reverse some of the damage that's occurred.

In addition to preventing cardiovascular disease, the steps outlined in this chapter are critical to treating heart disease and preserving heart function. Remember, you have far more control over your heart health than you may realize.

few pounds can significantly reduce many of these damaging effects. Losing just 5% to 10% of your body weight can lower your risk of cardiovascular disease.

Make sleep a priority

Sleep is fundamental to good health, including cardiovascular health. An abundance of evidence supports the importance of adequate rest for the health of your heart and blood vessels.

Disrupted sleep leads to changes in blood pressure. Variability in how long you sleep or when you go to sleep — in other words, not following a regular sleep schedule — is associated with high blood pressure, abnormal cholesterol levels and diabetes-related insulin resistance. In addition, too little sleep has been linked to increased risk of heart attack. According to some estimates, getting just one additional hour of sleep a night can decrease that risk by 20%. The link between inadequate sleep and cardiovascular disease likely also has to do with chronic inflammation, which poor sleep tends to promote.

What's a good night's sleep? Getting enough uninterrupted sleep so that you wake up feeling rested.

Manage stress

Stress causes your blood pressure and heart rate to increase and your heart to contract more forcefully. It also promotes inflammation in the arteries that supply blood to your heart. Reducing your risk of cardiovascular disease involves learning to manage stress.

In today's world, there's no shortage of stressors, and most people feel they experience too much stress. The good news is that you can learn to tackle stress by engaging in daily habits that keep stress from becoming overwhelming.

Several therapies and approaches can help you control stress, including relaxation therapies, positive self-talk, spirituality and practicing daily gratitude. You can read more about these in Chapter 16.

Exercise also can be an effective tool for managing stress. Physical activity helps burn off stress-related tension. And if you exercise with a partner, you'll also enjoy social support. Another strategy in managing stress is avoiding situations and events that tend to trigger stress. So is carving out time each day for those things you enjoy doing — activities that bring you pleasure and comfort and that release pent-up energy.

YOUR LUNGS

As discussed earlier in this chapter, your heart and your lungs work hand in hand. Your veins collect oxygen-depleted blood and waste, such as carbon dioxide, from your body and return it to the right side of your heart. From there, it's sent it to your lungs via a large blood vessel called the pulmonary artery.

In your lungs, blood makes its way to approximately 300 million tiny elastic air sacs called alveoli. In the alveoli, carbon dioxide is removed from your blood, and oxygen added to it. This oxygen-rich blood is then sent back to the left side of your heart and is pumped throughout your body to fuel your cells.

Your lungs are soft and spongy. They expand to draw in air, and they contract to expel air. This is done with the help of your diaphragm, a strong wall of muscle that separates your chest cavity from your abdomen. Your ribs support and protect your lungs, heart and chest cavity. They move slightly to help your lungs expand and contract as you breathe.

Age-related changes

Similar to other parts of your body, your lungs change over time. They continue to develop during childhood and adolescence and fully mature during young adulthood. After about age 35, lung function tends to slowly decline. This can happen for several reasons.

Unlike what occurs in your heart and blood vessels, where tissues gradually become stiffer as you age, the opposite takes place in your lungs. Instead of stiffening, the lungs gradually become more flimsy (more compliant).

This happens because the millions of tiny alveoli in the lungs, along with other structures that help keep your airways open, become less elastic and lose their shape. The result is that getting air out of your lungs becomes more difficult. Your diaphragm also can weaken over time, decreasing your ability to fully inhale. These changes can cause you to feel short of breath (dyspnea). You may not notice it unless you're exercising.

In addition to the structural changes that occur in the lungs, nerves in lung airways that trigger coughing to get rid of foreign particles can become less sensitive, causing the particles to build up in the lungs. This can potentially block airways and damage lung tissue. Your immune system also may weaken (see Chapter 8), leaving your lungs more vulnerable to infection.

CONDITIONS THAT AREN'T TYPICAL

Not all changes in your lungs are ominous indications of disease. Don't worry if you run out of breath a little more easily while swimming or hiking than you did in your younger years. By the same token, you don't want to overlook signs and symptoms that might indicate a more significant problem. Lung conditions that can affect older adults include:

Infection

Your respiratory system has several defense mechanisms that prevent foreign materials and organisms from entering your lungs. When material enters the lungs and can't be forced out — through either forceful coughing or "sweeping" particles out by way of small structures called cilia — your immune system works to fight infections that may develop.

Sometimes, the body's mechanisms that trigger coughing, clear mucus or fight infection can weaken. If bacteria, viruses or fungi (such as mold) enter the lungs and become established there, they can cause several illnesses, from the common cold to more serious infections such as influenza, pneumonia and COVID-19.

Factors that can damage your lungs and place you at higher risk of lung infection include smoking and exposure to certain chemicals, pollutants and toxic fumes, including secondhand smoke. Additional factors that may increase your risk of infection include being over age 65, having a weakened immune system, having another lung disorder (such as asthma or COPD), and being significantly overweight.

Viruses that cause infections, such as the common cold, influenza and severe acute respiratory syndrome coronavirus 2 (COVID-19), generally travel through the air in the form of tiny droplets. The droplets are created when someone with an infection coughs, sneezes or talks. You may inhale the droplets directly, or you can pick up the germs from an object — such as a telephone or computer keyboard — and then transfer them to your eyes, nose or mouth.

Most people with a respiratory infection experience mild to moderate symptoms, but these common infections can cause severe medical complications and lead to death in some individuals.

Older adults and people with existing medical conditions are at greater risk of becoming seriously ill with respiratory infections such as influenza and COVID-19.

Common symptoms of a respiratory infection may include fever and tiredness. The virus can also cause shortness of breath, muscle aches, chills, sore throat, a cough runny nose, headache, digestive issues and rash. Serious complications may include:

- Difficulty breathing.
- Pale, gray or blue-colored skin, lips or nail beds — depending on skin color.
- Ongoing dizziness.
- Chest pain.
- Severe weakness or muscle pain.
- Dehydration.
- Additional viral and bacterial infections.

An annual flu shot can reduce your risk of influenza. Vaccination against COVID-19, including follow-up booster doses, may prevent you from getting the virus or keep you from becoming seriously ill if you're exposed to it. Talk to your health care provider about when you should receive the pneumonia vaccine, based on latest guidelines.

Other steps that you can take to reduce your risk of a respiratory infection include wearing a mask in public spaces, avoiding crowds and indoor places with poor ventilation, washing your hands often with soap and water and using hand sanitizer that contains at least 60% alcohol.

For more on immunizations, see pages 274-275.

COPD

Chronic obstructive pulmonary disease (COPD) is the overall term for a group of chronic lung conditions that obstruct lung airways, often due to inflammation that causes scarring of lung tissues and narrowing of passageways that carry air from tiny alveoli to the mouth. COPD tends to develop gradually and produces few symptoms in its early stages.

COPD is most often seen in current or former smokers, with 8 out of 10 COPD-related deaths related to smoking. It also may result from occupations associated with exposure to chemical fumes or dusts, such as from grain, cotton, wood or coal. Air pollution and toxic gases in the environment, such as smog, also can contribute to the disease.

The most crucial step in preventing infection and COPD, along with other lung diseases, is addressing risk factors early. Quitting smoking early in life can nearly normalize your lifetime risk of COPD and quitting even after 15 or more years of smoking can reduce your risk of COPD by more than 50%.

It's always a good idea to talk to your health care provider about your individual risk of lung disease and lifestyle changes that can prevent or slow deterioration of lung function.

If you want a true assessment of your lung health, you can take a spirometry test. This is a simple test in which you blow hard into a tube. The test can help your doctor understand your pulmonary function, especially if you're at risk of lung disease. If, for example, you're 40 years old and the test shows you're breathing at 75% of your predicted vital capacity, you may want to take protective measures to help improve your lung function or prevent further decline.

Asthma

Asthma is a condition in which your airways narrow and swell and may produce extra mucus. This can make breathing difficult and trigger coughing, a whistling sound (wheezing) when you breathe out and shortness of breath.

For some people, asthma is a minor nuisance. For others, it can be a major problem that interferes with daily activities and may lead to a life-threatening asthma attack. Asthma signs and symptoms include shortness of breath, chest tightness or pain, wheezing, trouble sleeping and coughing or wheezing attacks that are worsened by a respiratory virus.

It isn't clear why some people get asthma and others don't, but it's probably due to a combination of environmental and inherited (genetic) factors.

The number of adults age 65 and older who have asthma is about the same as the general population. Some older adults first developed the condition in childhood, while others were diagnosed as adults. Several factors can increase your chances of experiencing asthma, such as:

- Having a blood relative with asthma, such as a parent or sibling.
- Having another allergic condition, such as hay fever or atopic dermatitis.
- Being overweight.
- Being a smoker or being exposed to secondhand smoke.
- Exposure to exhaust fumes or other types of pollution.
- Exposure to occupational triggers, such as chemicals used in farming, hairdressing and manufacturing.

RESPONDING TO YOUR RISKS

There are several ways to help protect your lungs and maintain better lung function throughout your life. You can learn more about healthy lifestyle changes and how to incorporate them into your daily routine in Part 2.

- **Don't smoke.** Smoking damages your lungs and will accelerate and worsen the natural effects of aging.
- **Pay attention to air pollution.** Indoor and outdoor air pollutants can damage your lungs. Secondhand smoke, outdoor air pollution, chemicals in the home and workplace, and exposure to radon all may trigger or worsen lung disease. Take steps to keep the air around you clean and wear a mask when necessary.
- **Exercise.** Regular exercise is very important to good lung health. Exercise helps to keep your chest muscles strong, thereby improving your breathing.
- **Aim for a healthy weight.** Too much fat around your abdomen can interfere with your diaphragm's ability to fully expand your lungs. If you're overweight, a combination of exercise and healthy eating will double the benefit to your lungs.
- **Get regular checkups.** Seeing your doctor regularly can help prevent diseases, even when you're feeling well. This is especially true for lung disease, which sometimes goes undetected until it's serious. There are medications that can reduce lung

inflammation and prevent chronic airway remodeling. They're most beneficial when taken in early stages of disease.

- **Stay up to date with your immunizations.** To help prevent lung infections, get an annual flu shot, pneumonia vaccine if you're eligible, and your COVID-19 vaccine and boosters. See Chapter 17 for more on recommended vaccinations.

5

Your bones, muscles and joints

The human musculoskeletal system is a marvel of mechanics. Composed of bones, muscles, ligaments and tendons, it allows you to move in a myriad of ways. Until the system breaks down, as a result of an accident, disease or general wear and tear over time, it's easy to take everyday movement for granted. Being able to move freely and comfortably is a cornerstone to staying independent.

Whether you have retirement dreams of hiking mountains and rafting rivers or simply enjoying walks in the park and playing with your grandchildren, understanding how to safeguard your musculoskeletal health can help you make those dreams reality.

Most adults become less mobile with age. Maintaining your mobility as you get older is critical in preserving your health and independence so that you can actively enjoy your later years.

BONE BASICS

Bones are living, changing tissues. Bone's basic structure, its inner framework, is a mesh of fibers composed primarily of the protein collagen. Within this framework are deposits of minerals such as calcium and phosphorous, with smaller amounts of sodium, magnesium and potassium. These minerals mix with water to form a hard, cementlike substance that makes bone firm and gives it strength.

The hard outer layer of bone, called cortical bone, is covered by a thin membrane (periosteum) that contains blood vessels that supply nutrients to bone, as well as nerves that send pain messages to the brain in case of injury or disease.

The spongy inner layer of bone (cancellous bone) includes a type of tissue called bone marrow. Bone marrow is a soft substance that fills the holes and passageways in the interior portion of your bones. Bone marrow manufactures vital oxygen-carrying red blood cells, germ-fighting white blood cells and clot-producing platelets. In younger individuals, bone marrow is mostly red marrow, owing to its production of red blood cells. As we age, the red marrow gets replaced by yellow marrow, reflecting the presence of more fatty tissue.

Bone remodeling

Think of the bones that form your skeleton as a never-ending home repair project. Throughout your lifetime, bone is continuously removed and replaced by new bone in a process called bone remodeling. On a regular basis, millions of tiny sections on the surface of your bones are simultaneously under construction.

Bone remodeling occurs for several important reasons. One is simply to repair damage caused by wear and tear. Another is to ensure that enough calcium and other minerals circulate through the bloodstream to carry out bodily functions that depend on these minerals. Finally, remodeling occurs in response to physical activity. Your skeleton adapts to heavier loads and greater stress by forming new bone.

This skeletal regeneration occurs in two basic stages. The initial stage is bone breakdown (resorption), and the second is bone formation. As tends to be true with most remodeling projects, the demolition stage generally goes faster than the reconstruction phase. To maintain your skeleton, fewer sections are being broken down than are being rebuilt. For an individual age 35, about 1% of the skeleton is undergoing bone breakdown, while about 4% is undergoing bone formation. At that pace, your skeleton undergoes complete regeneration about every 8 to 10 years.

Bone density

In your younger years, your skeleton grows to keep pace with developments of childhood, adolescence and young adulthood. During this time, your bones grow larger, denser and stronger, and your bone mass increases. Bone mass, what's often referred to as bone density, typically reaches its maximum — known as peak bone density — in your late 20s or early 30s.

KEY BONE BUILDERS

Similar to vitamins, minerals are substances that your body needs in certain amounts for normal growth and function. Because your body can't manufacture most minerals and vitamins, you need to get them from the foods you eat or, in some cases, from supplements.

Minerals serve many important functions in your body, including the development and maintenance of bone. Bone serves as storage — like a bank — for certain minerals, including calcium, phosphorus and magnesium. When minerals such as these are lacking in your diet, they're extracted from the reserves in your bones. Heavy withdrawals from your bone bank, such as those that occur during pregnancy or prolonged bed rest or immobilization, can impair your skeleton's ability to function normally.

Calcium is the most important mineral for bone health. Almost all of your body's total calcium is stored in your skeleton. Besides keeping your bones and teeth strong, calcium is needed for your heart, muscles and nerves to function properly and for your blood to clot normally.

Additional minerals that contribute to bone health and maintenance are phosphorus and magnesium and trace amounts of a few others. Most people who eat a balanced diet or who take a standard multivitamin with minerals get sufficient amounts of these minerals.

Peak bone density varies from one person to another. It's influenced by:

- **Heredity.** Genetic factors account for about 75% of the variation in peak bone density among individuals.
- **Sex.** Peak bone density is generally higher in men than it is in women because men's bones are larger.
- **Race and ethnicity.** White people and people of Asian descent generally have a lower bone density than do people of Black, Latino or Native American descent.
- **Diet.** People who consume adequate amounts of calcium and vitamin D generally reach a higher peak bone density than do individuals who don't get enough calcium and vitamin D. Vitamin D is needed for your body to effectively absorb calcium.
- **Physical activity.** Exercise and activity, especially weight-bearing exercises, are positive skeletal influences because your bones respond to physical activity by becoming denser and stronger.
- **Hormone production.** Estrogen, testosterone and other hormones contribute to bone formation and the maintenance of your skeleton.
- **Lifestyle.** Smoking and excessive alcohol use have an adverse effect on bone density.
- **Chronic health conditions.** Health conditions associated with chronic inflammation, such as rheumatoid arthritis, can lead to reduced bone density.

COMMON AGE-RELATED CHANGES

As with other systems in your body, not all bone-related changes are indications of disease. Don't worry if you've lost a bit of height or if you wake up feeling a little stiff in the morning. At the same time, be aware of signs and symptoms that might indicate a more significant problem.

With age, the rate of bone breakdown begins to overtake the rate of bone formation, and the number of reabsorption sites increases. Because of these changes, your bone density gradually decreases, and your bones become more porous and brittle, putting you at increased risk of fractures.

The transition from bone maintenance to bone loss is slow. In a decade, you'll likely experience about 3% to 5% loss of bone. After menopause, bone loss speeds up dramatically in women. The acceleration is primarily due to decreasing levels of the hormone estrogen.

In addition to a decline in bone density, with time the gel-like disks located between the bones (vertebrae) that make up your spine often lose fluid and become thinner. Vertebrae also lose some of their mineral content, making each bone thinner. A common consequence of this is that you might lose some of your height. The average person loses 1½ to 3 inches in height over a lifetime.

Thinning of the disks in your spine can also cause weakness of the muscles that help you maintain a straight posture. As a result, you may stand and sit less straight than in your younger years. While a slight to moderate change in posture is common with age, development of a severely hunched or "humped" posture (hyperkyphosis) isn't a normal consequence of aging.

Another change in bone with age is the development of what are commonly referred to as bone spurs. Bone spurs are bony projections that develop along bone edges. Bone spurs often form where bones meet each other in your joints. They can also form on the bones of your spine. Most bone spurs cause no signs or symptoms. You might not realize you have bone spurs until an X-ray for another condition reveals the growths. In some cases, though, bone spurs can cause pain and loss of motion in your joints.

CONDITIONS THAT AREN'T TYPICAL

The most common bone disease to affect older adults is osteoporosis. It occurs when your body loses too much bone, makes too little bone or both. As a result, your bones become weaker, more brittle and prone to fracture. People with osteoporosis are more likely to break bones, most often in the hip, forearm, wrist and spine. Most hip, wrist and forearm fractures tend to be the result of falls or other trauma. Until recently, osteoporosis was considered a natural part of aging. But there's nothing natural about it.

The good news is that osteoporosis is as preventable as it is common. The keys to avoiding the disease are building a strong skeleton when you're young and slowing the rate of bone loss as you age.

Osteoporosis risk factors

A number of factors can increase the likelihood that you'll develop osteoporosis — including your age, race and lifestyle choices, along with certain medical conditions and treatments. Some of these factors are out of your control, while others you have the power to influence. Unmodifiable risk factors include the following:

- **Sex.** Fractures from osteoporosis are about twice as common in women as in men. But by age 70, women and men lose bone mass at about the same rate.
- **Age.** Your bones become weaker as you age. By the time a woman reaches her 70s or 80s, she may have lost up to a third of her bone mass. A man, meanwhile, may lose up to 20% of his bone mass.
- **Race.** You're at the greatest risk of osteoporosis if you're white or of Asian descent.
- **Family history.** Having a parent or sibling with osteoporosis puts you at greater risk.
- **Body frame size.** People who are exceptionally thin or have small body frames are at higher risk because they have smaller skeletons and therefore less bone mass.
- **Lifetime exposure to estrogen.** The greater your lifetime exposure to the hormone estrogen, the lower your risk of osteoporosis. Women have a higher risk of osteoporosis if they experienced early menopause or began menstruating later than average.

Risk factors for osteoporosis that you can control include the following:
- **Inadequate calcium and vitamin D.** Not getting enough of these bone-building nutrients, especially when young, lowers your peak bone mass and increases your risk of fractures later in life.
- **Other hormone problems.** Treatments for prostate cancer that reduce testosterone levels in men and treatments for breast cancer that reduce estrogen levels in women can accelerate bone loss. Similarly, too much thyroid hormone can cause bone loss. Osteoporosis also is associated with overactive adrenal and parathyroid glands (hyperparathyroidism).
- **Eating disorder.** Severely restricting food intake and being underweight weakens bone in women and men.
- **Sedentary lifestyle.** People who spend a lot of time sitting or lying have a higher risk of osteoporosis than do people who are more active. Bone health begins in childhood. The most physically active children often grow up to have greater bone density.
- **Excessive alcohol consumption.** Too much alcohol reduces bone formation and interferes with the body's ability to absorb calcium.
- **Tobacco use.** The exact role tobacco plays in the development of osteoporosis isn't clear, but tobacco has been shown to contribute to weak bones.
- **Medications.** Long-term use of steroid medications damages bone. Excess thyroid hormone to treat an underactive thyroid (hypothyroidism) can also cause bone loss. Some diuretic

medications can cause your kidneys to excrete more calcium. Long-term use of the blood-thinning medication heparin, the drug methotrexate, some antiseizure medications and aluminum-containing antacids can accelerate bone loss. The list of medications associated with bone loss is long. Regularly review your medications with your health care provider to see if you may be at risk of low bone-mineral density and osteoporosis.

WHAT YOU CAN DO

It's never too late to fight back against osteoporosis and other bone-related changes. Good nutrition, regular exercise and other healthy habits and behaviors are essential for keeping your bones healthy throughout your life.

Get enough calcium

Men and women between the ages of 18 and 50 need 1,000 milligrams (mg) of calcium a day. This daily amount increases to 1,200 mg when women turn 50 and men turn 70. Younger individuals who are still growing require more than 1,000 mg daily, and pregnant women require up to 1,500 mg a day. Good sources of calcium include:

- Low-fat dairy products.
- Dark green leafy vegetables.
- Canned salmon or sardines with bones.
- Soy products, such as tofu.
- Calcium-fortified cereals and orange juice.

If you find it difficult to get enough calcium from your diet, consider taking calcium supplements. But make sure not to take too much, to avoid other health problems. The Health and Medicine Division of the National Academies of Sciences, Engineering, and Medicine recommends that total calcium intake, from supplements and diet combined, shouldn't exceed 2,000 mg daily for people older than age 50.

Don't forget vitamin D

Vitamin D improves the body's ability to absorb calcium and improves bone health in other ways. You can get some of your vitamin D from sunlight. However, be aware that the sun protection factor (SPF) in sunscreen can interfere with the synthesis of vitamin D in the skin, blocking or reducing the amount of vitamin D acquired from sunlight.

Dietary sources of vitamin D include cod liver oil, trout and salmon. But because we don't consume large enough quantities of these foods, they can't be our sole source of vitamin D. That's why foods such as milk, cereal and some orange juices are vitamin D-fortified.

Most people need at least 600 international units (IU) of vitamin D a day. The recommendation increases to 800 IU a day after age 70. People without other sources of vitamin D, and especially with limited sun exposure, might need a supplement. Most multivitamin products contain between 600 and 800 IU of vitamin D. Up to 4,000 IU of vitamin D a day is safe for most adults.

Increase bone strength with exercise

Exercise can help build strong bones and slow bone loss. Exercise will benefit your bones no matter what your age, but you'll gain the most benefits if you start exercising regularly when you're young and continue to exercise throughout your life.

To build bone and reduce your risk of a fall, you want to combine strength-training exercises with weight-bearing and balance exercises. Strength training helps strengthen muscles and bones in your arms and upper spine. Weight-bearing exercises — exercises in which you're on your feet supporting your weight so that your weight is working against gravity — include walking, jogging, running, stair climbing, skipping rope, skiing and many impact-producing sports. They affect mainly the bones in your legs, hips and lower spine. Balance exercises such as tai chi can reduce your risk of falling, especially as you get older.

Shifting your exercise routine to be more focused on strength training and weight bearing as you age can set you up for better musculoskeletal health. Try to do these exercises at least two times a week. If you don't love hitting the free weights or weight machines at the gym, get creative. This could mean walking with free weights or using your own body weight, such as when doing squats or pushups, or doing some yoga exercises. Wearing a weighted vest while walking may also benefit your spine, provided the weights are symmetrically placed in the vest and the total amount of weight used is gradually increased.

In addition to activities that strengthen your bones, you also want to include those that help strengthen your back muscles and improve your posture. Good balance is crucial to preventing falls, and good posture may limit an excessively curved back.

You can learn more about exercises for good bone health in Chapter 14.

Don't smoke, and limit alcohol

If you smoke, talk to your health care provider about ways to quit tobacco use. If you drink alcohol, limit consumption to no more than one drink a day if you're a woman no more than two drinks a day if you're a man.

Discuss medications with your health care provider

If you're at risk of osteoporosis, medications may be prescribed to help prevent the disease. You may be a candidate for medication if you have low bone density but not enough bone loss to qualify as osteoporosis (what's called osteopenia), if you're at risk of a fracture or if you're taking a medication known to reduce bone density.

SHOULD YOU HAVE A BONE DENSITY TEST?

A bone density test is used to determine if you have bone loss and if the amount of bone loss is consistent with osteoporosis. The test uses X-rays to measure how many grams of calcium and other bone minerals are packed into a segment of bone. Bones most commonly tested are those in the spine and hips and sometimes the forearms.

Most healthy young people don't need a bone density test. But as you age, your risk of osteoporosis increases. This is especially true in women. If you're a postmenopausal woman, a bone density test is recommended. Even if testing reveals your bone health is good, this test can be a baseline measurement for future testing.

For men who haven't experienced fractures, the answer isn't quite as clear. The U.S. Preventive Services Task Force doesn't recommend routine bone density testing for men. Because men have a higher bone mass and lose bone more slowly than women, they're at a lower risk of fracture. However, men with multiple risk factors, including medications known to reduce bone density, should be screened for bone loss.

YOUR MUSCLES AND JOINTS

Muscle health is extremely important to longevity and quality of life in your later years. Strong muscles allow us to perform daily tasks of living and maintain our independence. There's also some evidence that good muscle health can lead to improvements in other organ systems. A key aspect of healthy aging is building and maintaining adequate muscle mass.

Your body contains some 650 muscles that primarily help you to move. Muscles are made of large cells, called fibers, that can contract, enabling them to shorten and lengthen, producing movement. Tendons connect your skeletal muscles to bone, and ligaments connect bones to bones.

Skeletal (striated) muscles help hold your skeleton together, give your body shape, and assist with voluntary movements

Your doctor may recommend a bone density test, regardless of sex, if you've:

- **Lost significant height.** People who have lost at least 1½ inches in height may have silent compression fractures in their spines. Osteoporosis is a common cause of this.
- **Fractured a bone.** Fragility fractures occur when a bone becomes so fragile that it breaks much more easily than expected. Fragility fractures can even result from a strong cough or sneeze. Most often, though, they occur due to falls from a standing position.
- **Taken certain drugs.** Long-term use of steroid medications, such as prednisone, interferes with the bone-rebuilding process — which can lead to osteoporosis.
- **Experienced a decline in hormone levels.** In addition to the natural drop in hormones that occurs after menopause, cancer treatments, such as those for breast cancer and prostate cancer, can increase the risk of osteoporosis.
- **Developed hypercalcemia.** This is a condition in which the parathyroid gland becomes overactive, causing the leaching of calcium stored in bone.

that you can control, such as walking and chewing. Smooth (involuntary) muscles, meanwhile, are automatically controlled by your nervous system and include functions such as forcing blood through the walls of the stomach to control digestion and helping to maintain blood pressure.

Skeletal muscles support joint structures, along with tendons and ligaments. A joint is a point where two bones make contact. Some joints are covered with cartilage, a rubbery tissue that helps to encourage movement and that absorbs some of the shock or weight involved in movement. Joints also contain fluid to facilitate motion.

COMMON AGE-RELATED CHANGES

Similar to what happens with your bones, you're likely to experience changes in muscle mass and joint function as you age.

Muscle mass

Most of us will lose approximately 30% of our muscle mass over our lifetimes. This loss generally begins in our early 40s and continues throughout life. The number and size of muscle fibers also decrease. Due to loss of muscle, you may find that some tasks become a bit more difficult in your 50s than they were in your 20s. As one example, handgrip strength decreases, making it more difficult to do things such as open a jar.

Interestingly, researchers are finding that loss of muscle mass and muscle strength has as much to do with inactivity as it does with age. The less active you are, the more you may notice muscular changes and the more difficulty you may have performing day-to-day activities. Unfortunately, 60% of Americans are insufficiently active or overtly inactive.

Loss of muscle also affects your metabolism. Skeletal muscle — the largest organ by weight in the human body — is a very important metabolic organ. Most of the carbohydrates that you consume during the day are transferred to your muscles in the form of a simple sugar (glucose). The sugar remains in muscle in its stored form, called glycogen. Glycogen is used as a fuel supply to support movement and physical activity and to maintain and repair fibers within muscle tissues. The high metabolic activity of muscle makes it a major determinant in how much energy (calories) you expend during the day, including while at rest. Loss of muscle mass means less energy expended — fewer calories burned.

A reduction in muscle mass and less physical activity are major factors in why adults tend to put on weight later in life. All of this means that maintaining muscle mass is incredibly important as you get older.

Joint flexibility and function

Muscles, tendons and joints lose flexibility with time. The water content of tendons decreases as you get older. This makes these movable tissues stiffer and less able to tolerate stress. In addition, the cartilage lining your joints may become thinner, and your joint surfaces may not slide over each other as smoothly as they used to. All of these changes are why you may not be able to perform certain movements as easily as you once did, such as take a seated position on the floor, swing a golf club or bend down to tie your shoes.

Osteoarthritis

Osteoarthritis is a very common condition and one of the leading causes of disability. More than 50 million Americans have some form of the disease.

Osteoarthritis — often simply called arthritis — results when cartilage, the slippery, lubricating substance that normally cushions the ends of bones, breaks down. This breakdown causes the lining in a joint (synovium) to become inflamed, further damaging the cartilage. As the ends of the bones become exposed, they thicken and form bony growths, resulting in pain from bone rubbing against bone.

Osteoarthritis can affect any joint in your body. It may strike only one joint, such as a knee or a hip. Or it may involve multiple joints, such as those in your fingers. In addition to pain, reduced mobility in a joint is a principal feature of the disease.

Nearly two-thirds of people with osteoarthritis are under age 65, and symptoms often begin after age 40. Nevertheless, the risk of getting the disease increases as you get older.

Risk factors

Wear and tear is the most common cause of osteoarthritis, but the disease can occur for several reasons. Other factors that increase your risk include:
- **Age.** Osteoarthritis becomes more common with age.
- **Sex.** Of people older than age 65 who have osteoarthritis, 75% are women.

- **Certain hereditary conditions.** Some people are born with defective cartilage or slight defects in how their joints fit together. With age, these defects can cause early cartilage breakdown.
- **Joint injury.** If you've injured a joint due to sports, work-related activity or an accident, you may be at increased risk of developing osteoarthritis — especially of the knees.
- **Obesity.** Excess weight puts unnecessary pressure on your spine, knees and hips and can lead to osteoarthritis.
- **Other medical conditions.** Diseases that change the normal structure and function of cartilage also can increase your risk of developing osteoarthritis.

CONDITIONS THAT AREN'T TYPICAL

Even though the body's musculoskeletal system is extremely durable, muscle and joint injuries are common. A fall or an accident can overstretch muscles or extend a joint beyond its normal range of motion. Wear and tear on your body's muscles and joints can lead to injury.

Back pain is a common complaint. When you think of all the work that your back does each day — constantly bending and twisting as you go about your day-to-day activities — it's not surprising that problems develop. It's estimated that more than 80% of American adults will experience at least one bout of back pain during their lifetimes.

It's normal to feel some back pain as you age, usually beginning between ages 40 and 60. And the older you are, the more likely your chances of encountering a bout of back pain or developing a back-related disorder.

Because back pain is so common, you may think that it's inevitable — it's not. Certain factors put you at greater risk. They include tobacco use, being overweight, being inactive and experiencing stress, anxiety or depression. A physically demanding job — especially one involving heavy lifting, unbalanced bending or repeated actions — may increase your risk. Finally, and not surprisingly, age and years of wear and tear on your muscles, ligaments and bones can increase your risk.

Causes of back pain

Conditions that are commonly linked to back pain include:
- **Muscle or ligament strain.** Repeated heavy lifting or a sudden awkward movement can strain back muscles and spinal ligaments. For individuals in

poor physical condition, constant strain on the back can cause painful muscle spasms.

- **Bulging disks.** Disks act as cushions between bones in the spine. The spongy, gel-like material inside a disk can bulge, which can irritate the nerves in your spine and cause significant back pain. Bulging disks can affect more than one vertebra in the spine and can become degenerative if not treated. Bulging disks don't always

RHEUMATOID ARTHRITIS: IT'S NOT THE SAME AS OSTEOARTHRITIS

Rheumatoid arthritis causes painful aching and swelling in your joints and is one of the most debilitating forms of arthritis. Unlike osteoarthritis, which generally results from years of wear and tear, rheumatoid arthritis is an autoimmune disorder. It develops when your immune system mistakenly attacks the tissue (synovium) that lines your joints. Also, unlike osteoarthritis, rheumatoid arthritis isn't more common with age.

Rheumatoid arthritis often occurs at a younger age than osteoarthritis typically does, and it affects three times more women than it does men. In contrast to osteoarthritis, which affects primarily bones and cartilage, rheumatoid arthritis can target your whole body. It can affect organs that you might not expect, such as your heart, lungs and eyes. However, the disease most commonly affects the joints.

Scientists don't know exactly what causes the immune reaction that leads to rheumatoid arthritis, but certain factors may increase risk of the disease. They include certain genes, an infection, hormonal influences and smoking. People who are overweight also appear to be at a somewhat increased risk of developing rheumatoid arthritis.

Treatment mainly involves medications to control inflammation and pain and to slow joint damage.

cause back pain; disk disease is often found on imaging tests performed for another reason.

- **Ruptured disks.** A disk that ruptures is generally a result of an injury. Ruptured disks are usually limited to a single location (vertebral level) and can occur at all ages.
- **Arthritis.** Osteoarthritis can affect the lower back. In some cases, arthritis in the spine can lead to a narrowing of the space around the spinal cord, a condition called spinal stenosis. Morning back stiffness that lasts for less than 30 minutes may be associated with osteoarthritis. Morning stiffness lasting longer than 30 minutes may be a result of other rheumatological conditions.
- **Osteoporosis.** The bones (vertebrae) that make up the spine can develop painful breaks if they become porous and brittle.
- **Spinal stenosis.** It results when spaces in the spine narrow, placing pressure on the spinal cord and nerve roots. The condition most often occurs in the lower back and neck and is often due to wear and tear related to arthritis.

WHAT YOU CAN DO

Early intervention is the key to staving off conditions that can affect your muscles and joints. By adopting healthy lifestyle habits early on, it may be possible to keep your joints flexible and your muscles strong. Following are steps that can improve the health of your joints and muscles. You can read more about many of them in Part 2.

Aim for a healthy body weight

Excess weight places added stress on joints in your back, hips, knees and feet, and it strains your back muscles. The best way to achieve and maintain a healthy weight is with regular exercise and a healthy diet.

Develop a sustainable activity program

It's important to follow a well-rounded activity plan to maintain muscle strength throughout your body, including your spine, and range of motion in your joints. An activity plan can also help you manage conditions such as osteoarthritis and back pain. For these conditions, a health care professional, such as a physical therapist, can tailor the proper program to meet your needs.

Your weekly workout should include aerobic exercise, strength training, balance exercises, and flexibility exercises.

To gain the most benefit from an activity program, aim for 150 minutes a week of moderate-intensity activities or 75 minutes a week of more vigorous exercise.

Low-impact aerobic activities increase muscle strength and endurance and allow your muscles to work better. Walking, bicycling and swimming are good choices. Strength training exercises provide joint support, and they build muscle, including your core abdominal muscles that support your back. Balance exercises help improve your posture and coordination, as well as your core strength. Flexibility exercises improve range of motion in your joints and surrounding muscles.

Explore mind-body practices

Mind-body practices such as yoga and tai chi reduce tension in your muscles and improve strength, flexibility and balance. They're beneficial for your overall health, including your musculoskeletal health.

Yoga combines physical poses with controlled breathing and meditation or relaxation. Tai chi is a graceful form of exercise that involves a series of movements performed in a slow, focused manner and accompanied by deep breathing. Studies have shown both practices to be helpful in maintaining overall well-being, including muscle and joint health.

Eat well to maintain a healthy weight

To achieve a healthy weight and reap the benefits of good nutrition, follow a diet that emphasizes vegetables and fruit, whole grains, low-fat dairy, lean meats and/or plant-based proteins and healthy fats, such as nuts and olive oil.

Get enough sleep and manage stress

A restful night allows your brain and body, including your back and your joints, to recover from the day's activities and challenges. Too much stress affects your overall health and may cause you to tense your muscles. This tension can contribute to back problems. Stress may also cause you to overeat or not exercise, making it more difficult to maintain a healthy weight.

Wear the right shoes

Buy and wear comfortable shoes that properly support your weight. This is especially important in preserving the health of your weight-bearing joints and your back.

Maintain good posture

As you go about your day, your posture is probably the last thing on your mind. But the way you stand, sit and lift can make a big difference when it comes to your musculoskeletal health, especially your back health. Poor posture causes uneven weight distribution and may strain your ligaments and muscles. To maintain your posture, practice the following:

- **Stand smart.** Don't slouch. When standing for long periods, place one foot on a low footstool to take some of the load off your lower back. Alternate feet. Good posture can reduce the stress on back muscles.
- **Sit smart.** Choose a seat with good lower-back support, armrests and a swivel base. Change positions frequently, at least every half hour.
- **Lift smart.** Avoid heavy lifting, if possible. If you must lift something heavy, let your legs do the work. Keep your back straight — no twisting — and bend only at the knees. Hold the load close to your body. Find a lifting partner if the object is heavy or awkward.

WHAT DO YOU THINK?

As you reflect on what you just read and contemplate your future health, ask yourself these questions.

- *How do I feel about my current musculoskeletal health?*
- *What am I doing now that I feel good about?*
- *What are some aspects of my musculoskeletal health I'd like to improve?*
- *What changes can I make that I'm most likely to stick with?*

Your digestive health

6

Digestion is one of the critical functions your body must perform to survive and thrive. The food you eat and the beverages you drink provide necessary nutrients that supply your cells with sustenance and energy so that your body can develop, maintain and repair itself.

How your digestive system works may seem easy to understand. You put food in your mouth. Your digestive organs break down the food. Nutrients in the food are absorbed in your intestines. The rest is eliminated as waste.

Sounds pretty simple, doesn't it? In fact, the human digestive system is incredibly complex. Sometimes things can go wrong, and over time the process may become less efficient.

With age, your body's intricate process of gathering nutrients and removing waste and liquids starts to change in many ways, some that you can't control. But there are steps you can take to help keep your digestive system healthy.

YOUR TEETH AND MOUTH

How your teeth and gums respond to age depends on how well you've cared for them over the years. But even if you're meticulous about brushing and flossing, you may still notice that your mouth feels drier than when you were younger, which could be related to medications you take or your diet. With age, your gums may also recede, and your teeth may darken slightly and become more brittle.

Tooth loss can be a challenge for older adults, but the good news is that over the past two decades, the oral health of Americans has significantly improved. Older adults are having fewer teeth extracted, and fewer people need dentures because better attention is being paid to preventive dental care, including improved treatments for gum disease. Additionally, as fewer people use tobacco than in past generations, more older adults are keeping their teeth.

Seeing a dentist regularly and following recommended practices are keys to preventing tooth loss and maintaining good oral health.

Conditions that aren't typical

While understanding that changes to your teeth and mouth are common with age, you don't want to overlook signs and symptoms of more significant problems. Your oral health can contribute to various diseases and conditions, including:

Gum disease

Gingivitis is a common and mild form of gum disease that causes irritation, redness and swelling (inflammation) of your gingiva, the part of your gum around the base of your teeth. It's important to take gingivitis seriously and treat it promptly. It can lead to a more serious gum disease called periodontitis and tooth loss. Gum disease may be an indicator of widespread chronic inflammation, a possible predictor for cardiovascular disease. Some studies suggest that individuals with gum disease may be at twice the risk of heart attack and stroke.

Healthy gums are firm and pale pink and fitted tightly around the teeth. Signs and symptoms of gingivitis include swollen, puffy or dusky red gums; gums that bleed easily when you brush or floss; significantly receding gums and bad breath.

The most common cause of gingivitis is poor oral hygiene that encourages plaque to form on teeth, causing inflammation of the surrounding gum tissues.

Gum disease also appears to be more frequent and severe among people who have diabetes. And research shows that people with gum disease have a harder time controlling their blood sugar levels.

Dry mouth

Dry mouth refers to a condition in which the salivary glands in your mouth don't make enough saliva to keep your mouth wet. A dry mouth can make speaking, swallowing and tasting more difficult. It was once thought that dry mouth was a normal part of aging, but we now know that it can be related to other causes such as medications. Hundreds of common medications, including pain-killers, allergy medications, blood pressure drugs and antidepressants can lead to dry mouth. Certain health conditions may also cause dry mouth, such as Sjogren's syndrome, autoimmune disease, yeast infections (thrush) and diabetes insipidus.

Having adequate saliva is important. Saliva helps prevent tooth decay by neutralizing acids produced by bacteria, limiting bacterial growth and washing away food particles. Saliva also enhances your ability to taste and makes it easier to chew and swallow. In addition, enzymes in saliva aid in digestion.

What you can do

Most dental and oral diseases are preventable and treatable at every age.

- **Brush your teeth at least twice a day.** Brush your teeth on all sides with a soft-bristled toothbrush and fluoride toothpaste. Be sure to clean the outer and inner surfaces of your teeth and gums.
- **Floss daily.** Careful flossing will keep your gums healthy by removing plaque and food that a toothbrush can't reach. Rinse after you floss. If you have trouble handling floss with your fingers, a floss holder can help.
- **Rinse.** Use mouthwash to remove food particles left after brushing and flossing.
- **Visit your dentist regularly.** See a dentist at least once a year for a professional cleaning and checkup. Your dentist will check for cavities, gum disease and oral cancer.
- **Avoid tobacco products.** Tobacco used in any form, including cigars, pipes and chewing tobacco, increases the risk of gum disease and oral and throat cancers.

YOUR DIGESTIVE TRACT

It's normal for digestion to change as you age. With time, muscles in the digestive tract tend to become stiffer and weaker. The stomach becomes less elastic and can't hold as much food. Digested food moves more slowly through your intestines. And the amount of surface area within your intestines diminishes slightly, so that the small intestine may be less able to absorb certain nutrients.

The flow of secretions from your stomach, liver, pancreas and small intestine may also decrease. The liver may become smaller, and the enzymes it produces may work less effectively. As a result, it may take longer to rid your body of medications and other substances. This means the effects of drugs can last longer.

In addition, over time, acid levels in your gut may decrease, the enzymes that break down food may evolve and the bacteria that naturally reside in your large intestine may change, all making you more susceptible to digestive issues.

Your gut microbiome and your health

You've likely heard the saying, "You are what you eat." We've known for many years that what we put into our bodies can affect our health. But as science has evolved, it's becoming clearer that our health may also be defined by the trillions of microorganisms that live inside us.

In various parts of our bodies — in the mouth, skin, vaginal or respiratory tract, for example — reside a wide variety of microorganisms. But nowhere are these microorganisms greater in number and diversity than in the gastrointestinal system, commonly referred to as the gut. Diversity refers to how many different species of microorganisms are in your stomach and how evenly distributed they are. Diversity is crucial, as it's a hallmark of a healthy gut.

Most of the time, your gut contains the right kind and the right amounts of microorganisms that communicate with almost every area of your body and help you maintain good overall health. But sometimes the balance of these microorganisms can be disrupted, causing a reduction in good bacteria and an increase in potentially harmful bacteria. A gut imbalance is thought to play some part in the development of several diseases and disorders.

Over the last several years, much information has been published on the gut microbiome, looking at all aspects of the subject. This is due, in part, to improved testing that can better analyze the microbiome. Researchers continue to explore how a gut imbalance may be associated with the development of disease, from conditions that probably aren't so surprising, such as digestive disorders, to those you may not expect, such as autism.

Early beginnings

Your gut microbiome is the total environment of your gut — not only specific microorganisms and their genetic components but also their surroundings. Think of it as an ecosystem; much like the ecosystem of Iceland varies from that of Brazil, so, too, does the environment of the gut vary from one person to another.

The formation of this microbial ecosystem begins early on. Research suggests that prior to being born, our digestive tracts are almost like a blank slate. After birth, many outside influences begin to help shape the microbiome.

For example, an infant born via vaginal delivery will have gut bacteria that differs from an infant born via cesarean section. This is because the mother passes along bacteria to her child during a vaginal delivery. Babies who are breast-fed will have a different gut makeup from babies who consume formula. By the time a child is a toddler, the child will have gut microbiota as diverse as an adult's. All told, our bodies house about 100 trillion gut microorganisms, including several hundred different species of bacteria.

For the most part, your gut microbiota remain stable. But certain factors can alter it — for example, medications or a change in diet. Aging can have an impact because the microbiota tend to become less diverse as we get older. Taking antibiotics can also disrupt healthy flora. This increases the chances of conditions that result from decreased diversity in the gut, such as C. diff. (Clostridioides difficile) infections. An imbalance may also be linked to other gastrointestinal illnesses, such as irritable bowel syndrome, as well as allergies, obesity and neurological issues.

Nurturing a healthy gut

The science involving the gut microbiome isn't at the point yet where researchers can definitively determine if an unbalanced gut microbiome causes disease or if a disease or the medications used to treat it are to blame. They do know, though, that certain foods and lifestyle habits seem to help promote gut health. For example, moderate to vigorously intense aerobic exercise has been shown to improve the composition of microbiota in your gut.

Research also suggests that eating plant-based foods, such as whole grains, fruits and vegetables, and peas and beans (legumes) supply good bacteria to our gastrointestinal system. These foods contain complex carbohydrates. Our bodies can't digest complex carbohydrates, so they become food for gut bacteria, allowing them to thrive. Foods that contain active cultures, such as yogurt, kimchi and kombucha, also may provide helpful bacteria.

In addition, increasing evidence suggests our gut microbiome influences more than just our digestive health. It influences overall health, and having a healthy gut may actually increase longevity.

In the future, we may be able to tailor our diets to cultivate desirable gut microbiota. Until that day, the best strategy is to exercise and eat a balanced diet to keep your gut happy. It's also important to pay attention to the use of antibiotics. Only take them when prescribed by a health care provider, so they don't upset the delicate balance of gut microbiota through overuse.

COMMON AGE-RELATED CHANGES

Digestive changes with age are often so subtle that you may not notice them. But they commonly occur. Some people experience more bloating and acid reflux or become less tolerant of certain kinds of food. Others have issues with constipation or metabolizing medications.

Some common digestive-related conditions occurring with age include the following.

Occasional heartburn

Heartburn — that burning pain in the chest that usually occurs after eating — is often more noticeable and common as you get older. The reason for this is that our digestive muscles become less responsive. As food is transported into the stomach, it passes through the lower esophageal sphincter, the muscle that controls the opening between the esophagus and the stomach. Over time, contraction of this muscle can become weaker, allowing stomach contents to return (reflux) into the esophagus.

Occasional heartburn is common. However, frequent heartburn is often associated with a condition called gastroesophageal reflux disease (GERD).

THE GUT-BRAIN CONNECTION

Have you ever had a gut-wrenching experience or felt the butterflies in your stomach? Most people have. That's because the body's brain and gastrointestinal system are intimately connected, and they "talk" to each other a lot. This link between those cells that control your digestive functions and those that regulate your brain's emotional center is called the gut-brain axis.

Increased disease and disability that come with age can trigger feelings of stress and anxiety, causing greater communication between your brain and gut. What this means in regard to digestion is that when you're anxious, worried or feeling stressed, you don't digest food well. Not surprisingly, a lot of gastrointestinal disorders are associated with stress and anxiety.

When you're under stress, your body reacts as if you're in danger. It pumps extra blood to your muscles so that you'll have more energy to fight off an attack or to run away. This leaves less blood volume to support digestion. Your digestive muscles exert less effort, your body secretes fewer enzymes to aid digestion and the passage of food and waste through your digestive tract shifts into low gear. This produces symptoms such as heartburn, bloating and constipation.

Sometimes stress does the opposite. It speeds passage of food through your intestines, causing abdominal pain and diarrhea. Stress may also worsen symptoms of digestive conditions such as ulcers, irritable bowel syndrome and ulcerative colitis.

Other brain-related conditions can affect your gut. It's not uncommon for people who are depressed or anxious to lose their appetites and, as a result, lose weight. Additionally, people with anxiety issues tend to experience more problems with diarrhea or GERD. This is why caring for your mental health can improve your digestive health.

Less tolerance for lactose

Among some individuals, as they get older their bodies produce less lactase, an enzyme needed to digest the sugar (lactose) in milk. This may result in some difficulty digesting dairy products. Normally, lactase turns milk sugar into two simple sugars, glucose and galactose, which are absorbed into the bloodstream through the intestinal lining. You can have low levels of lactase and still be able to digest milk products. But if your levels are too low, you become lactose intolerant.

More difficulty with bowel movements

As undigested food waste moves more slowly through the colon, more water gets absorbed from the waste and stool becomes drier, leading to constipation. Many other factors can exacerbate the problem, such as medications or supplements, including calcium and iron supplements. Lack of physical activity and not drinking enough fluids are generally the most common culprits. Other factors include a diet low in fiber, changes to your diet, illness and putting off bowel movements. Overuse of laxatives, especially fiber-based ones, can lead to chronic constipation if not taken with adequate amounts of water.

CONDITIONS THAT AREN'T TYPICAL

While some changes to your digestive health may be an inevitable part of aging, don't overlook signs and symptoms of more significant problems. Millions of Americans experience some type of digestive issue. Evidence of this is on display in drugstore and grocery store aisles lined with an impressive array of digestive-related medications and supplements. If your symptoms are more than mild and occasional, discuss them with your health care provider.

Chronic constipation

One of the most common digestive complaints among older adults is constipation. Passage of stools becomes less frequent and may be difficult and painful. When symptoms of constipation last for several months, it's considered chronic constipation. Chronic constipation is thought to affect up to 20% of adults in the United States, with more women reporting the problem than men. The condition becomes more common with age, affecting up to one-third of individuals age 65 and older.

Constipation is generally described as having fewer than three bowel movements a week, but symptoms vary. There are many causes for this condition, including too little liquid, too little dietary fiber and too little activity. Medications and other medical conditions such as pelvic floor problems, prior surgeries or radiation to the bowels also can lead to the problem.

Dietary and lifestyle changes often can help prevent or treat chronic constipation. If these measures aren't enough, a number of medications are available to help treat the problem.

Chronic diarrhea

Diarrhea results when the lining of your intestines becomes inflamed, hampering their ability to absorb nutrients and fluids. Often diarrhea is related to an infection or consumption of a particular food and is short-lived, but sometimes it can become chronic.

Chronic diarrhea may be related to diseases that cause inflammation or to conditions such as malabsorption and hypermotility. A common cause of chronic diarrhea is irritable bowel syndrome.

Sometimes, the problem is related to undigested sugars. If this is the culprit, it's best to avoid so-called FODMAP carbohydrates, including dairy-based foods; wheat-based products; beans and lentils; some vegetables, including asparagus, onions and garlic; and some fruits, including apples, cherries, pears and peaches. Chronic diarrhea may also stem from an intolerance or sensitivity to other foods or food components. Excessive consumption of caffeine or alcoholic beverages can cause chronic diarrhea, as can certain medications.

Dietary and lifestyle changes may help relieve some chronic diarrhea. If the problem is related to an inflammatory illness, medication may be necessary to treat it.

Lactose intolerance

Food intolerances and *food sensitivities* are terms used to describe signs and symptoms that develop when a person has difficulty digesting a particular component of food. This can lead to problems such as gas, abdominal pain or diarrhea. There are several types of food intolerances. One of the most common is lactose intolerance.

As mentioned previously, individuals who are intolerant to lactose have difficulty digesting the sugar (lactose) in dairy products because their bodies don't produce enough of the enzyme lactase. When lactose isn't absorbed, it travels to the colon, where fermentation takes place. During fermentation, bacteria convert the lactose to gas and fluid, causing cramping, diarrhea, bloating and gas.

Lactose intolerance varies. Most people have no problem consuming small amounts of dairy products. Their signs and symptoms occur when consuming several dairy products at once or eating a large portion of food containing lactose. People with more severe intolerance can't eat any dairy products without experiencing distressing symptoms.

There's no way to boost your body's production of lactase. The best way to manage lactose intolerance is to avoid those foods that cause problems and use lactose enzyme products when consuming dairy foods. These products break down lactose so it can be absorbed.

Cultured or fermented dairy products such as yogurt and cheese contain the least amount of lactose because the culturing process predigests much of the lactose. Most of the lactose in dairy is associated with the whey, which is removed in the making of hard cheeses. So the longer a cheese is aged and the harder it is, the less likely it contains lactose. Goat cheese also tends to be lower in lactose.

GERD

Nearly everyone experiences heartburn on occasion — that hot, burning sensation in your chest, and sometimes your throat, caused by stomach acid washing back into your esophagus. Occasional heartburn is generally nothing to worry about, but in some people stomach acid reflux occurs frequently, even daily.

Constant backwash of stomach acid can damage tissues of the esophagus. This can lead to formation of scar tissue, which may narrow the esophagus and make swallowing more difficult. Gastroesophageal reflux disease (GERD) also increases the risk of esophageal cancer.

Anyone can develop GERD, but certain factors place you at greater risk. They include being obese, having a hiatal hernia and being pregnant. Other factors can aggravate acid reflux, including:
• Smoking.
• Eating large meals or eating late at night.
• Eating certain foods (triggers) such as fatty or fried foods.

- Drinking certain beverages, such as alcohol or coffee.
- Taking certain medications, such as aspirin.

Maintaining a healthy weight can help prevent acid reflux or reduce its frequency. It's also helpful to wait at least three hours after eating before lying down or going to bed and to limit or avoid foods that can trigger reflux. Common triggers include alcohol, chocolate, caffeine, fatty foods and peppermint.

And if you smoke, quit. Smoking decreases the ability of the lower esophageal sphincter, the muscle that controls the opening between the esophagus and the stomach, to function properly.

RESPONDING TO YOUR RISKS

It's clear that what you put on your plate has a lot to do with good digestion. But it's not only what you eat that's important. How much you eat and the manner in which you eat — relaxed or hurried, focused or distracted — also play key roles.

Your daily food choices and eating habits can go a long way toward keeping your digestive system strong and healthy. Of course, you can't prevent or manage all digestive problems simply by following a healthy lifestyle. Some digestive disorders are hereditary or occur for unknown reasons.

Many digestive problems, however, can be prevented or relieved by adopting a healthier diet, eating slowly, managing stress and engaging in regular physical activity. If you can stick with these changes, gradually they become habits. Those habits, in turn, become a routine, and eventually that routine becomes your new lifestyle. The benefits are many. In addition to improving your digestive health, healthier habits can reduce your risk of disease and help you look and feel better.

Focus on fiber and nutrients

Make sure to eat plenty of fruits, vegetables and whole grains. These foods are rich in nutrients, including dietary fiber. Fiber is an important part of a healthy diet and is especially important to digestion.

Adequate fiber in your diet can prevent constipation and reduce your risk of other digestive disorders such as hemorrhoids. Fiber also helps encourage the growth of healthy and diverse bacteria in your gut.

Fiber is the part of plant food that's indigestible and that your body doesn't absorb. Fiber comes in two forms, soluble and insoluble, and fiber-rich foods usually contain both forms. Soluble fiber gives food bulk and it absorbs a lot of water as it moves through your digestive tract. Insoluble fiber, meanwhile, helps speed up the transit of food in the digestive tract and helps prevent constipation by keeping waste moving.

ANOREXIA OF AGING

As people age, many tend to eat smaller meals and eat more slowly due to digestive changes. As a result, some people see a reduction in their daily calories of up to 25%.

If you're trying to lose weight, this natural occurrence may be a cause for celebration, especially since maintaining a healthy weight is such a focus of health. For some people, though, a reduction in calories can lead to unintended weight loss in which they become underweight, known as the anorexia of aging.

While it doesn't receive much attention, anorexia of aging can become a serious problem. It often results in inadequate nutrition, can affect muscle strength and energy level and can lead to frailty (see Chapter 11).

On occasion, anorexia of aging may point to an underlying disease or social challenge. Sometimes it can signify alcoholism, emotional problems such as depression, and late-life paranoia or cognitive impairment. With age, some individuals worry that eating too much will harm them or they simply forget to eat. Anorexia in a person's later years may also suggest an undiagnosed malignancy, dental or swallowing problems or lack of help with shopping and cooking.

If you have difficulty maintaining healthy weight or feel that you're losing too much weight, talk with your health care provider.

NEED TO ADD MORE FIBER TO YOUR DIET?

Here's a look at how much dietary fiber is found in some common foods. Women should try to consume at least 21 to 25 grams of fiber a day, and men should aim for 30 to 38 grams daily.

Food	Serving size	Total fiber (grams)*
Split peas, boiled	1 cup	16.0
Lentils, boiled	1 cup	15.5
Black beans, boiled	1 cup	15.0
Baked beans, canned	1 cup	10.0
Chia seeds	1 ounce	10.0
Green beans, boiled	1 cup	9.0
Raspberries	1 cup	8.0
Spaghetti, whole-wheat, cooked	1 cup	6.0
Barley, pearled, cooked	1 cup	6.0
Pear	1 medium	5.5
Bran flakes	¾ cup	5.5
Broccoli, boiled	1 cup chopped	5.0
Quinoa, cooked	1 cup	5.0
Oat bran muffin	1 medium	5.0
Oatmeal, instant, cooked	1 cup	5.0
Apple, with skin	1 medium	4.5
Brussels sprouts, boiled	1 cup	4.0
Potato, with skin, baked	1 medium	4.0

*Rounded to the nearest 0.5 gram.

Source: USDA National Nutrient Database for Standard Reference, Legacy Release.

Also, make sure you're getting the recommended amounts of vitamins and minerals.

Include foods containing probiotics

Probiotics are often referred to as friendly bacteria or good bacteria. They're beneficial microorganisms that facilitate the fermentation process. Foods containing probiotics are thought to be good for your digestive system because they contain good microbes that help combat and crowd out any bad bacteria that may be lurking in your gut. Probiotic foods may help reduce diarrhea and constipation and promote overall gut health.

Probiotics can be found in yogurt that contains active or live cultures. Yogurt is made by fermenting milk with different bacteria, which are left in the final product. Other sources of probiotics include some cheeses, sauerkraut, a fermented milk drink called kefir, Korean fermented vegetables known as kimchi, and kombucha, a tea.

Drink plenty of fluids

Along with a high-fiber diet, fluids can help prevent digestive problems by allowing waste to pass more easily through the digestive tract. Try to drink 64 ounces of fluid daily — that's eight 8-ounce glasses of fluid daily. Water is the best. And remember that most vegetables and fruits are at least 80% water.

How much fluid you need depends on a variety of factors, including your health, where you live, how active you are and how much you perspire. For some people, fewer than eight glasses might be adequate. Others might need more fluid — for example, if you have a history of kidney stones or renal insufficiency. Also keep in mind that if you have a specific medical condition, such as heart disease, you may need to limit your fluid intake. If you're uncertain how much fluid you should consume, discuss it with your health care provider.

To help make it easier to keep track of how much water you drink, you might purchase a 1-liter water bottle, and make sure you drink at least two bottles of water a day. Two liters is roughly equivalent to 64 ounces.

Try not to skip breakfast

Morning is one of the best times of day to take advantage of regular muscle contractions taking place within your colon, known as gastrocolic reflex. This reflex helps move waste from the colon to the rectum, triggering an urge to expel stool.

Eating breakfast loads your digestive system with food — and ultimately food waste — helping promote regular bowel movements. When you sense a pending bowel movement, go to the bathroom right away. Delaying bathroom use can contribute to constipation.

Limit your portions

Large meals increase demand on your digestive system. Your body is able to produce only a certain amount of digestive juices, and if you eat too much, not enough juices may be available to meet the task. This can increase your risk of heartburn. Moderate proportions, meanwhile, are digested more comfortably. Plus, eating smaller portions can help maintain a healthy weight.

Eat at regular times

Your digestive system operates best when you follow a regular schedule — such as eating three meals a day instead of eating whenever you feel like it. With a regular schedule, your digestive system has time to rest between meals.

Don't rush your meals

Hectic schedules can leave you rushing through your meals or eating on the go. When you eat fast, you often overeat before your stomach can signal that it's full — which leads to overconsumption and weight gain. In addition, you tend not to chew your food long enough or not to grind it into small enough pieces, forcing your digestive system to work harder. When you gulp down food rapidly, you swallow more air than you would if you were eating slowly. This can lead to belching, bloating and intestinal gas.

To make sure food digests properly and stomach acid doesn't regurgitate into your esophagus, don't eat while lying down. And don't lie down right after a meal. Wait at least three hours after eating before lying down or going to bed.

Keep physically active

Physical activity is very important to digestion. It helps speed the movement of food through your digestive tract, keeping your bowels moving and promoting regularity. In addition, exercise can help you maintain a healthy weight.

For more information on exercise and developing an exercise program, see Chapter 14.

7

Your urinary health

As you read in the previous chapter, when you eat and drink, your body breaks down what you consume into substances that are absorbed into your bloodstream. As your blood circulates, your body's cells absorb liquid and nutrients from your blood and deposit wastes back into it. The job of your urinary system is to remove, collect, store and eliminate excess fluid and waste from your blood through urination.

Your urinary system includes the kidneys, the long muscular tubes (ureters) that carry urine from the kidneys to your bladder, the bladder and the slender drainage tube (urethra) that carries urine from your bladder out of your body. Urinary problems aren't a normal part of aging but can become more frequent as you get older.

COMMON AGE-RELATED CHANGES

Around age 40, your kidneys begin to lose essential filtering units called nephrons. This loss can cause you to lose some kidney function. Among other things, you may become dehydrated more quickly and retain fluid more easily.

In as many as one-third of healthy adults, however, kidney function remains unchanged with age.

The kidneys have a built-in reserve capacity, and despite the loss of nephrons they continue to function normally. If you have a chronic illness, such as high blood pressure or diabetes, kidney changes can pose a greater risk and may require adjustments to your medications.

The bladder also changes with age. Its walls become less elastic, so it isn't able to hold as much urine as it used to. This is why you may find yourself needing to go to the bathroom more often. Over time, the bladder's muscles can weaken and may contract more frequently.

One result of these changes is that your bladder may leak more easily. Another is that your bladder may not completely empty when you go to the bathroom, which can increase the risk of urinary tract infections (UTIs).

CONDITIONS THAT AREN'T TYPICAL

Minor urinary changes generally aren't a problem, but more severe changes can lead to illness and interfere with daily living. The following urinary conditions are often seen more commonly with age.

Urinary tract infections (UTIs)

People generally become more vulnerable to UTIs as they get older. This is often related to weakening of muscles in the bladder and in the pelvic floor that can lead to urine retention or urine leakage. Whenever urine stays in the urinary tract, there's a potential for bacteria, such as Escherichia coli (E. coli), to multiply and cause an infection.

UTIs are more common in women than in men because the female anatomy makes it easier for bacteria to enter the urinary tract. Women also experience UTIs more frequently after menopause, when estrogen levels decrease. The loss of estrogen can alter the pH of the vagina, making it less acidic, which in turn makes it easier for bad bacteria to grow. Reduced estrogen may also lead to general thinning of the vaginal wall and increased inflammation and irritation of urinary tissues. With age, especially after menopause, the tissues of the urethra and bladder become drier, increasing the risk of irritation and infection. Among men, an enlarged prostate gland can increase the risk of UTIs.

UTIs often can be prevented or reduced by staying hydrated, following good bathroom and hygiene habits and addressing factors that may place you at higher risk of infection.

Urinary incontinence

Despite what you may think or have been told, loss of bladder control (urinary incontinence) isn't a normal part of aging. But incontinence becomes more common as you get older. The problem affects both men and women but is more common in women. The reasons why are much the same as for urinary tract infections — loss of muscle support, thinning and drying out of tissues and reduced estrogen levels (in women).

Women who've had multiple vaginal childbirths or who are obese may be at greater risk of stress incontinence. Stress incontinence refers to urine leakage that results from exerting pressure (stress) on the bladder by coughing, sneezing, exercising or lifting something heavy.

Among men, noncancerous (benign) prostate gland enlargement, prostate cancer and prostate surgery are common causes of incontinence. Other factors contributing to incontinence in both men and women include infections, excess weight, frequent constipation and a chronic cough.

Certain drinks, foods and medications may act as diuretics, stimulating your bladder and increasing urine volume, increasing the risk of bladder leakage. They include alcohol, caffeine, carbonated drinks, artificial sweeteners, chocolate, highly spiced foods and several medications, including some used for depression, high blood pressure and heart disease. Constipation and tobacco use also are risk factors for incontinence.

The good news is that urinary incontinence often is manageable with the right treatment, and in some cases may be preventable. Strategies that can help decrease your risk include maintaining a healthy weight, practicing pelvic floor muscle exercises, avoiding bladder irritants, eating more fiber to prevent constipation and quitting smoking.

Chronic kidney disease

This condition, also called chronic kidney failure, involves a gradual loss of kidney function. Your kidneys filter wastes and excess fluids from your blood, which are then removed in your urine. As the kidneys fail, waste builds up. Advanced chronic kidney disease can cause dangerous levels of fluid, electrolytes and wastes to accumulate in the body.

BLADDER IRRITANTS

The following foods and beverages are associated with bladder irritability. Some of them affect the bladder by making urine more acidic. Others, such as spicy foods, can inflame the lining of the bladder. And foods containing caffeine may irritate bladder tissues as well as lead to involuntary bladder contractions associated with urge incontinence — a sudden, intense urge to urinate, followed by involuntary loss of urine.

It's not necessary to avoid all the items listed here. But if some of them seem to be causing you problems, you may want to reduce how much you consume or stay away from them all together.

Carbonated beverages
- Soda
- Sparkling water

Alcohol
- Beer
- Liquor
- Wine, wine coolers

Caffeine
- Coffee
- Tea
- Chocolate

Citrus fruits and juices
- Oranges
- Grapefruit
- Lemons

- Limes
- Mangos
- Pineapple

Tomatoes and tomato-based foods
- Tomato juice
- Tomato sauce
- Barbeque sauce
- Chili

Onions and spicy foods
- Foods that use chili peppers or other pungent spices

Foods containing vinegar
- Pickled foods
- Dressings
- Some condiments

Products containing aspartame and saccharin
- Diet soda
- Sugar-free foods such as ice cream, cocoa mix and candy

Be aware that some vitamins, supplements and medications also contain ingredients such as caffeine, citrus juices and artificial sweeteners.

In its early stages, chronic kidney disease may produce few signs or symptoms. Because the kidneys can often make up for lost function, signs and symptoms may not become noticeable until the disease is advanced.

Loss of kidney function can cause a buildup of fluid or body waste or electrolyte problems. Depending on how severe the condition is, loss of kidney function may cause a variety of symptoms, including nausea and vomiting, loss of appetite, fatigue and weakness, urination changes and swelling of the feet and ankles.

Conditions that increase risk of chronic kidney disease include diabetes, high blood pressure, cardiovascular disease and obesity. Your risk is also increased if you smoke, have a family history of kidney disease, take medications that affect the kidneys, or are of Black, Native American or Asian ancestry.

Treatment for chronic kidney disease generally focuses on slowing the progression of kidney damage, usually by controlling its cause. But even controlling the cause might not keep kidney damage from progressing to end-stage kidney failure, which is fatal without artificial filtering (dialysis) or a kidney transplant.

Kidney stones

Kidney stones form when a change occurs in the normal balance of water, salts, minerals and other substances in urine. Higher than normal levels of calcium, oxalate and phosphorus in your urine can lead to the development of hard pebblelike pieces of material that vary in size.

About 11% of men and 6% of women in the United States experience kidney stones at least once during their lifetimes. The stones can develop in any part of your urinary tract, from your kidneys to your bladder. Often, they form when urine becomes concentrated, allowing minerals to crystallize.

Kidney stones generally have no definite, single cause, although several factors may increase your risk.

- **Family or personal history.** If someone in your family has had kidney stones, you're more likely to develop stones, too. If you've already had one or more kidney stones, you're at increased risk of developing another.
- **Dehydration.** Not drinking enough water each day can increase your risk of kidney stones. People who live in warm, dry climates and those who sweat a lot may be at higher risk than others.

- **Certain diets.** Eating a diet that's high in protein, sodium (salt) and sugar may increase your risk of some types of kidney stones. This is especially true with a high-sodium diet. Too much salt in your diet increases the amount of calcium your kidneys must filter and significantly increases your risk of kidney stones. Foods rich in compounds called oxalates — such as rhubarb, beets, okra, spinach, Swiss chard, sweet potatoes, nuts, tea, chocolate, black pepper and soy products — can increase your risk of other types of stones.
- **Obesity.** A high body mass index (BMI), a large waist size and weight gain have been linked to an increased risk of kidney stones.
- **Certain supplements and medications.** Vitamin C, dietary supplements, laxatives (when used excessively), calcium-based antacids and certain medications used to treat migraines or depression can increase your risk of kidney stones.

Benign prostatic hyperplasia (BPH)

Benign prostatic hyperplasia (BPH) — also called prostate gland enlargement — is a common condition for men as they get older. An enlarged prostate gland can cause uncomfortable urinary symptoms, such as a blockage of urine flow out of the bladder. It can also cause bladder, urinary tract or kidney problems.

After age 40, the male prostate gland — primarily the gland's transitional zone — begins to enlarge, which is sometimes referred to as a second growth spurt. It's estimated that nearly 70% of men from ages 60 to 70 and close to 90% of men older than age 80 have some degree of BPH.

As the gland enlarges, tissue within it often becomes lumpy, forming characteristically uneven cell mass clusters. Smooth muscle in the prostate reacts to this buildup by constricting and tightening around the urethra, narrowing the drainage channel and obstructing urine flow from the bladder.

The condition can be extremely disruptive for some men and pose few problems for others. Signs and symptoms of BPH vary in their severity and may include:

- A frequent or urgent need to urinate.
- Frequent urination at night (nocturia).
- Difficulty starting urination.
- A weak urine stream or a stream that stops and starts.
- Dribbling at the end of urination.
- An inability to completely empty the bladder.

The exact cause of prostate enlargement is unknown, and it's likely that several factors play a role in its development. In addition to age, family history can increase your odds of developing the disease, pointing to a possible genetic link. However, genetics is thought to play a role in only a small percentage of cases. There's some evidence that obesity may increase the risk of BPH, while exercise can lower it. And studies show that diabetes, as well as heart disease and medications called beta blockers, might increase BPH risk.

Steps that may reduce your risk of prostate enlargement and help catch the problem early include eating well, getting regular exercise and seeing your doctor regularly.

RESPONDING TO YOUR RISKS

Some factors that place you at increased risk of urinary problems, such as your age and your genes, are outside your control. But you do have control over other factors, such as your lifestyle habits.

Consume the right amount of fluid

Drinking too much fluid can make you urinate more frequently. But not drinking enough can lead to a concentration of waste in your urine, which can irritate the bladder. The daily fluid recommendation for adults is about 64 ounces, equal to approximately eight 8-ounce glasses or two 1-liter bottles.

If you're bothered by urinary tract infections, you might consider drinking cranberry juice as part of your daily fluid intake. Although research in this area is inconsistent, there is some evidence that cranberry juice may work to prevent recurrent infections.

Some people find that drinking this much fluid is a problem. They need to go to the bathroom all the time, including getting up several times at night to urinate. To help alleviate this, consider the following:

- Drink more of your fluids in the morning and afternoon rather than at night.
- Skip alcohol and beverages with caffeine, such as coffee, tea and cola, which increase urine production.
- Remember that fluids come not only from beverages but also from foods such as soup.

You might also try bladder training, also known as timed voiding. With bladder training, you go to the bathroom on a set schedule and gradually increase the time between urination. A bladder-training program usually follows these steps:

- **Identify your pattern.** For a few days, keep a diary in which you note every time you urinate.
- **Extend your urination intervals.** Using your diary, determine the amount of time between urinating. Then extend that by 15 minutes. If you usually urinate every hour, try to extend that to an hour and 15 minutes. Gradually lengthen the time between trips to the toilet until you reach intervals of 2 to 4 hours. Be sure to increase your time limit slowly to give yourself the best chance for success.
- **Stick to your schedule.** Once you've established a schedule, do your best to stick to it. Urinate immediately after you wake up in the morning. Thereafter, if an urge arises, but it's not time for you to go, try to wait it out. Distract yourself or use relaxation techniques such as deep breathing. If you feel you're going to have an accident, urinate but then return to your schedule.

Get enough fiber and limit sodium

Eating foods that are high in fiber — whole grains, legumes, fruits and vegetables — can help prevent constipation, which can contribute to incontinence. A healthy diet can also help you maintain a healthy weight, reducing the overall pressure on your bladder and the pelvic floor muscles that support it.

Studies show that a diet low in sodium, such as the Dietary Approaches to Stop Hypertension (DASH) diet, can reduce your risk of kidney stones. In addition to being low in sodium, DASH limits consumption of red meat and promotes fiber.

Keep active

Regular exercise is important for many reasons. It helps strengthen your pelvic floor muscles. It helps you maintain a healthy weight. And it may help prevent prostate enlargement. All of these are key to good urinary health. For more information on exercise, see Chapter 14.

Practice pelvic floor exercises

In both men and women, pelvic floor exercises, known as Kegels, can help treat mild to moderate incontinence and may help prevent it. To do the exercises, imagine that you're trying to stop urine flow or avoid passing gas in public. Squeeze the muscles you would use to do this for a count of five — if five is too long, start with three. Do this 10 times, resting between contractions. Repeat the exercises three or four times a day. To maintain the benefits, you'll need to keep doing them.

To be sure you're doing the exercises correctly, ask your health care provider for help or to refer you to a physical therapist knowledgeable about pelvic floor exercises.

Be cautious with medications

Medications are a common cause of urinary problems and can exacerbate existing conditions. Review all your medications with your provider. Individuals with kidney disease are generally advised not to take nonsteroidal anti-inflammatory drugs (NSAIDs), with the exception of aspirin, because they're associated with kidney injury and may worsen progression of the disease.

Over-the-counter decongestants and cold medications can tighten the muscles that control urine flow, making urination more difficult. And some prescription medications with anticholinergic properties — actions that interfere with certain brain neurotransmitters — may slow the release of urine from your bladder.

WHAT DO YOU THINK?

As you reflect on what you just read and contemplate your future health, ask yourself these questions.
- *How do I feel about my current urinary health?*
- *What am I doing now that I feel good about?*
- *What are some aspects of my urinary health I'd like to improve?*
- *What changes can I make that I'm most likely to stick with?*

Some high blood pressure and heart medications can relax bladder muscles, allowing urine to flow more easily and sometimes leak. Other medications, including diuretics, can trigger or worsen incontinence by causing you to produce more urine.

Stop smoking

Smokers are more likely to have bladder control problems and to have more severe symptoms. See your health care provider for help with quitting tobacco.

Your immune health

8

Keeping infectious microorganisms out of your body and destroying any that get in are key missions of your immune system. At one time, scientists had only fragments of information about how the various cells that make up the immune system interact to protect us against disease. But after decades of research, they now believe that more than 100 million immune cells exist.

For each harmful substance — a virus, bacterium, parasite, toxin — there is an immune system cell that is specially designed to seek out and destroy it.

Your body's immune system also plays a key role in helping to fight cancer. It actively patrols the body looking for cancerous cells and eliminates them as they arise.

This is the grounding principle behind an emerging field of medicine called cancer immunology. As researchers have sought to understand why the immune system sometimes fails to protect us from cancer, they've learned how to manipulate immune cells to make them more effective cancer fighters — a form of treatment called immunotherapy.

Another key function of the immune system is to mount an inflammatory response, such as in wound healing. When your skin is cut, punctured or scratched, specialized immune cells produce proteins that signal your skin to grow and reseal the injured site. These proteins trigger production of substances that protect the injured area from bacteria growth. In the case of a fractured bone, your immune system activates a chain of healing reactions to bridge the gap between the fractured sections and to repair the injury.

It comes as no surprise, then, that a critical component of good health is maintaining a healthy immune system. When your immune system is strong, your body is better prepared to fight off illness and repair itself. When your immune system is weaker, you're more likely to get sick. This is especially true as you get older, when your immune system tends to work less efficiently.

Fortunately, the body's immune system is very redundant, so that even in older age, it's still sufficiently functional in handling common encounters of daily living. However, the recent COVID-19 pandemic, in which most deaths occurred among individuals age 65 and older, serves as a reminder that the system is fragile.

IMMUNE BASICS

As you take steps to protect your immune health, you may find the following information about your immune system helpful to understand.

Innate vs. acquired immunity

There are two types of immune responses — innate immunity and acquired immunity. Innate immunity is the first response of your body's immune system to a foreign substance. When harmful substances, such as bacteria or viruses, enter the body, certain cells in the immune system quickly respond and try to destroy them. Innate immunity also includes barriers, such as skin, mucous membranes, tears and stomach acid, that help keep harmful substances from entering your body.

Acquired immunity refers to immunity that's not present at birth — immunity that your body learns. This type of immunity develops when your immune system responds to a foreign substance or microorganism or after you receive antibodies from another source.

There are two types of acquired immunity: adaptive and passive. Adaptive immunity occurs in response to being infected with or vaccinated against a microorganism. Your body produces an immune response, which can prevent future infection by the microorganism. Passive immunity occurs when you receive antibodies to a disease or toxin via injection rather than your own immune system making them.

Acute vs. chronic inflammation

Your body produces two types of inflammation: acute and chronic. Acute inflammation is the redness, warmth and swelling that result with an injury, such as when you cut yourself. Your immune system responds to the cut by releasing white blood cells to surround and protect the area. Acute inflammation helps your body fight infection and enables healing. The process works similarly if you have a cold or the flu. When you start to feel better, the inflammation goes away.

Chronic inflammation, meanwhile, is inflammation that lingers. It doesn't go away after a few days or weeks. This form of inflammation is thought to develop in response to chronic infection or tissue injury and may be aggravated by things such as an unhealthy diet, too little exercise, ongoing levels of high stress and environmental pollutants.

Other causes of chronic inflammation include persistent infections, autoimmune diseases and obesity. Instead of serving as a healing force, chronic inflammation becomes damaging, causing a variety of problems (see page 16).

COMMON AGE-RELATED CHANGES

As you get older, your immune system generally loses some of its strength. It doesn't operate as quickly or efficiently as when you were younger. Because of this, the following changes may occur.

Slower immune response

With age, your immune system isn't as fast at responding to threats, which can increase your risk of getting sick. Immune cells known as B and T cells located throughout your body continually look for harmful invaders (antigens). Over time, these cells decline in number and become less efficient at surveying for antigens. As a result, your body's ability to recognize new invaders decreases, and you become more susceptible to infections and other diseases and disorders.

If you become ill with an infection, you may experience fewer symptoms and lower fevers than in your younger years. A fever is a sign of a healthy immune response. A lower fever suggests your immune response is decreased. In addition, flu shots and other vaccines may not work as well or protect you for as long as they once did.

Slower healing

You may notice that it takes longer for an injury to heal than when you were younger. This is due in part to fewer immune cells circulating throughout your body to aid in healing efforts.

Reduced cellular repair

Part of what your immune system does is detect and correct damaged cells. This response also declines over time. Fewer repairs to damaged cells can place you at increased risk of various diseases, including cancer.

Increased risk of chronic inflammation

Over time, your body's immune cells can produce a low-grade, chronic inflammation. It's a sort of nagging inflammatory response that's unproductive — it doesn't fight anything. The effects of this unhealthy immune response can accumulate, harming healthy tissues and placing you at increased risk of disease.

CONDITIONS THAT AREN'T TYPICAL

It's important to understand that changes within your immune system are common with age. Similar to any type of aging army, over time your natural defenses can weaken and become less efficient at fending off invaders. But you don't want to overlook indications of more serious problems.

A significantly weakened immune response can make it difficult for your body to detect and react to serious threats to your health, placing you at increased risk of severe illness. And sometimes your immune system can overreact. For example, a person may experience an immune response even though there's no real threat. This can lead to problems such as allergies, asthma and autoimmune diseases.

As you age, your immune system may become less able to distinguish normal cells from foreign invaders (antigens). This is why autoimmune disorders typically become more common as you get older. If you have an autoimmune disease, your immune system attacks healthy cells in your body by mistake. There are more than 80 types of autoimmune diseases, which include conditions such as rheumatoid arthritis, psoriasis, inflammatory bowel disease and type 1 diabetes. Signs and symptoms of autoimmune disorders vary but often include fatigue, achy joints and muscles, swelling and redness, skin rashes, low-grade fever and difficulty concentrating. Each disease can have its own unique symptoms.

Over time, the body's immune system may become less able to detect and defend against cancer cells and subsequent tumor growth. When cancer cells show up in your body, your immune system usually kills them before they can form a tumor. But if your immune system is weakened, the abnormal cells are able to grow and form a tumor.

The good news is that novel treatments such as immunotherapy are revolutionizing cancer treatment by igniting the immune system's natural ability to clear cancerous cells from the body. For more information on cancer risks with age, see Chapter 10.

Other immune system problems occur when your immune system doesn't work correctly. This may be related to a genetic mutation, as in the case of immunodeficiency diseases, or it may be associated with damage to the system. For example, human immunodeficiency virus (HIV) harms the immune system by destroying white blood cells. If HIV isn't treated, it can lead to AIDS (acquired immunodeficiency syndrome) and increase risk of several other severe illnesses. COVID-19 is another example. Scientists and researchers are actively studying the effects of the SARS-CoV-2 virus on the immune system, especially in cases of severe disease. One researcher described an immune system afflicted by severe COVID-19 infection as going "immunologically haywire."

WHAT YOU CAN DO

A healthy lifestyle is your best weapon in keeping your immune system strong and reducing many of the risks associated with an aging immune response. A healthy lifestyle can also help prevent chronic inflammation, which places you at greater risk of several diseases, including cardiovascular disease, diabetes, Alzheimer's disease and cancer. Getting ahead of chronic inflammation in midlife is one of the best strategies to stave off its more detrimental effects as you age.

The basic tenets of a healthy lifestyle likely sound familiar: Exercise, eat well, maintain a healthy weight, don't smoke, limit alcohol, reduce stress and get enough sleep. (You can learn more about these lifestyle principles throughout this book.) For your immune health, it's also important to keep up to date on recommended vaccines, including your annual flu shot and the COVID-19 primary series and boosters (see Chapter 17).

Boost your immunity with exercise

Research has made it abundantly clear that exercise is good for your immune health. Exercising every day, such as taking a 30-minute walk, can help your body fight infection. If you don't exercise regularly, you're more likely to catch a cold, for example, than someone who does. Exercise also helps boost your body's feel-good chemicals (endorphins) and helps you sleep better, both of which are good for immune health.

Studies of older adults who are more active have found that in addition to other important health benefits, they tend to have better immunity. Studies also indicate that older individuals who participate in moderate strength training, endurance activities and high-intensity interval training generally experience reduced inflammation.

The key takeaway: Physical activity typically declines with age, so it's especially important to keep active as you get older.

Load up on fruits and vegetables

As with exercise, there's an abundance of research pointing to a healthy diet as a way to boost your immunity as you age. Nutritious foods help keep your immune system strong.

Fruits and vegetables are important to your immune health because they're rich in nutrients such as vitamins C and E, beta carotene and zinc. Try to eat a wide variety of brightly colored fruits and vegetables, such as berries, citrus fruits, kiwi, apples, red grapes, kale, onions, spinach, sweet potatoes and carrots. They contain high amounts of beta carotene, which converts into vitamin A.

It's best to get these key vitamins from eating healthy foods rather than from taking over-the-counter vitamins and supplements. If you have dietary limitations that prevent you from eating many vitamin-rich foods, talk to your health care provider or a registered dietitian about the best way to supplement the vitamins and minerals your diet is missing.

Other foods associated with immune health include leafy greens; fatty fish, which contain healthy omega-3 fatty acids; nuts and seeds; garlic and ginger; olive oil; and yogurt. Probiotic foods, such as yogurt with live cultures, encourage gut health, which appears to support a healthy immune system.

Another key step is to limit or avoid foods that promote chronic inflammation, such as fried foods, red and processed meats, unhealthy fats and foods high in sugar and refined carbohydrates. Sugar also curbs the action of immune system cells that attack bacteria. This effect occurs immediately after consuming sugar and can last a few hours or more.

In addition, a healthy diet contributes to a more active lifestyle, and as you just read, increased activity is good for your immune health. It also decreases your risk of obesity. This is important because studies indicate that obesity can result in an impaired immune response or impaired immune functioning, increasing the risk of infection and other immune-related problems.

Don't smoke, and limit alcohol

Many of the chemical compounds found in cigarette smoke can interfere with your immune system, causing it to work less effectively in fighting disease and infection and giving both the opportunity to progress. Similarly, excess alcohol may suppress a wide range of immune responses, making you more vulnerable to infection and disease and making it more difficult to recover from illness.

Pay attention to stress

Stress can be short-term (acute) or long-term (chronic), and its effects accumulate over time. Acute stress is a reaction to an immediate or perceived threat. When you experience or sense danger, such as an angry-looking dog, your brain sets off an alarm system known as your fight-or-flight response. This same reaction occurs in other stressful situations, such as speaking in front of a large audience.

During the fight-or-flight response, your body produces hormones, including adrenaline (epinephrine) and cortisol, that help it respond to the threat. Once the threat has passed, these hormone levels drop and your body returns to a normal, relaxed state.

Too much stress causes this fight-or-flight response to remain turned on, and this isn't good. The longer your stress response system is engaged, the more cortisol and other stress hormones are being produced. Too much cortisol can suppress the effectiveness of your immune system by reducing your body's white blood cells, which help fend off infection. This places you at greater risk for bacterial and viral infections, including those that cause colds and flu.

Taking steps to decrease stress in your life can help slow immune changes. Several mind-body practices such as yoga, meditation and progressive muscle relaxation can help you relax.

WHAT DO YOU THINK?

As you reflect on what you just read and contemplate your future health, ask yourself these questions.

- *How do I feel about my current immune health?*
- *What am I doing now that I feel good about?*
- *What are some aspects of my immune health I'd like to improve?*
- *What changes can I make that I'm most likely to stick with?*

Get enough sleep

It's become increasingly clear that sleep and the immune system are closely connected. Consistent sleep strengthens your immune system, allowing for balanced and effective immune function. Lack of sleep, on the other hand, can throw it off. Evidence indicates that both short- and long-term sleep deprivation can make you sick.

When you're tired, even from just one night of poor sleep, brain regulation of the immune system weakens, making you more susceptible to infections.

In addition to reduced risk of infection, healthy sleep habits are associated with better outcomes when you do get an infection and a better response to vaccinations. Sleep helps your immune system store information about infectious invaders, including mild ones introduced by a vaccine. This stored memory equips your immune system to recognize and block the germs the next time they come around. Lack of sleep, on the other hand, can reduce your immune response to vaccines by up to 20% to 25%.

CHAPTER 9

Weight, sleep, skin and sexual health

You've likely heard some version of the saying, "If you feel good, you look good." A need to feel good about our appearance is why stores are filled with products from anti-aging creams to hair dyes to weight-loss supplements. We all want to maintain a young appearance as we get older, but the reality is that with time, many aspects of our appearance do change, such as our skin, hair and weight.

What's important to remember is that your well-being isn't tied solely to your appearance; it's about how you feel. And if you feel good, you'll look good! So, even if your hair is getting grayer, your skin has a few more wrinkles and your body has lost some of its shape, that doesn't mean that you can't still look great. Feeling good about yourself is important because it affects your overall well-being, and your overall well-being has an impact on your physical health.

Personal well-being involves nurturing those things that help us feel good about ourselves. We discuss many of them in Part 2 of this book, including maintaining and building social connections, having purpose in life, eating well and getting regular exercise. Well-being also involves other aspects of daily living, such as sleep and sex. With age, some people find that good sleep and sexual relationships become more difficult, as a result of both hormonal and psychosocial changes. Sleep can help you live well and possibly longer. And the need for intimacy is ageless.

WEIGHT AND HEALTH

Obesity is a major health issue in the United States. Two-thirds of the adult population is overweight, and 1 in 3 adults is considered obese. With the easy availability of calorie-dense foods, the bombardment of commercial messages urging you to eat and the prevalence of sedentary work and leisure activities, it's easy to pack on pounds.

At a certain point, body fat can interfere with your health. The more your weight increases, the more problems you may face in staying healthy and living longer. And, as you may already know, preventing weight gain becomes more difficult as you age.

In clinical research studies, obesity — technically defined as having a body mass index of 30 or greater — has been repeatedly associated with an increased risk of heart disease, stroke, diabetes, certain cancers, digestive and liver problems, infertility, erectile dysfunction, sleep apnea and osteoarthritis. In fact, it's been connected to almost all modern illnesses that plague us. Obesity is also linked to a higher rate of premature death.

A healthy weight is important to a fulfilling, long life. The good news is that you can improve your weight without dieting. If you focus on the habits discussed in this book — a healthy diet, exercise, good sleep, social support and limited alcohol intake — your weight will likely improve. All of these habits put together can help you shed excess pounds, enjoy a more active, energetic life and reduce your risk of many diseases.

Age and weight

With age, we naturally tend to gain weight, to the tune of 1 to 2 pounds a year. That may not seem like much, but over time it can lead to significant weight gain and, in some cases, obesity. Not everyone becomes overweight as they age because body weight is influenced by a variety of factors, including genetic makeup, physical activity, and food choices. Still, most people find that with each passing year, maintaining or losing weight becomes more difficult.

WHAT'S YOUR BMI?

To determine your BMI, find your height in the left column. Follow that row across to the weight nearest yours. Look at the top of that column for your approximate BMI. Or use this formula:

1. Multiply your height (in inches) by your height (in inches).
2. Divide your weight (in pounds) by the results of the first step.
3. Multiply that answer by 703. (For example, a 270-pound person, 68 inches tall, has a BMI of 41.)

	Healthy		Overweight					Obese				
BMI	19	24	25	26	27	28	29	30	35	40	45	50
Height						Weight in pounds						
4'10"	91	115	119	124	129	134	138	143	167	191	215	239
4'11"	94	119	124	128	133	138	143	148	173	198	222	247
5'0"	97	123	128	133	138	143	148	153	179	204	230	255
5'1"	100	127	132	137	143	148	153	158	185	211	238	264
5'2"	104	131	136	142	147	153	158	164	191	218	246	273
5'3"	107	135	141	146	152	158	163	169	197	225	254	282
5'4"	110	140	145	151	157	163	169	174	204	232	262	291
5'5"	114	144	150	156	162	168	174	180	210	240	270	300
5'6"	118	148	155	161	167	173	179	186	216	247	278	309
5'7"	121	153	159	166	172	178	185	191	223	255	287	319
5'8"	125	158	164	171	177	184	190	197	230	262	295	328
5'9"	128	162	169	176	182	189	196	203	236	270	304	338
5'10"	132	167	174	181	188	195	202	209	243	278	313	348
5'11"	136	172	176	186	193	200	208	215	250	286	322	358
6'0"	140	177	184	191	199	206	213	221	258	294	331	368
6'1"	144	182	189	197	204	212	219	227	265	302	340	378
6'2"	148	186	194	202	210	218	225	233	272	311	350	389
6'3"	152	192	200	208	216	224	232	240	279	319	359	399
6'4"	156	197	205	213	221	230	238	246	287	328	369	410

Based on *Circulation*, 2014;129(suppl 2):S102; NHBLI Obesity Expert Panel, 2013.
*Asians with a BMI of 23 or higher may have an increased risk of health problems.

One reason we tend to gain weight over time is that the amount of lean muscle we have naturally begins to decline by about 3% to 8% per decade after we

IS A LITTLE EXTRA WEIGHT OK AS YOU AGE?

What's considered a healthy weight may be different for older and younger people. Studies indicate that current weight guidelines may be too restrictive for older adults. Researchers found that being moderately overweight may not be as risky to an older person's health as once thought and that a few extra pounds might help you live longer.

One study of more than 16,000 individuals age 65 and older found that men and women who were slightly overweight — who had a BMI range of 25 to 29.9 — had the lowest death (mortality) rate over a period of nine years. Mortality was higher in both men and women with BMIs below 25 — considered a healthy weight. Other studies have produced similar results.

The research has prompted a discussion about whether being a little overweight in your older years actually may be good for your health. The answer is, possibly. But keep in mind that in most studies, those individuals who were slightly overweight and who lived longer generally didn't have other weight-related health conditions, such as diabetes or osteoarthritis. And among older adults who were obese, not just slightly overweight, the results weren't the same. Studies generally reported increased mortality in obese older adults.

What all this means is that, no matter what your age, it's important to avoid obesity — a BMI of 30 or more — to prevent disease. By the same token, you don't want to be underweight. That, too, can be dangerous later in life. Aim for a happy medium. Once you reach your late 60s and 70s, if you're generally healthy, being slightly overweight may not be a risk to your health and might actually be protective.

after we enter our 30s. If you're less active because of a health condition or if you've been sidelined with an injury or surgery, you may also lose muscle.

Why does loss of muscle matter? Lean muscle, even muscle at rest, burns about five times more calories than does fat. A decrease in muscle mass is likely to slow your metabolism, a complex process that converts food calories into energy. Unless you regularly include strength training in your exercise routine to maintain and build muscle, your body will need fewer calories each day. If you continue to consume the same number of calories as you did when you were younger, you're likely to gain weight.

Another reason controlling your weight becomes more difficult as you get older is that both men and women undergo changes in hormone levels. In women, this happens at menopause, when levels of the hormone estrogen decline. Beginning around age 40, men gradually experience a drop in the hormone testosterone, at a rate of about 1% to 2% per year.

Testosterone and a form of estrogen called estradiol are responsible for, among other things, regulating metabolism. With fewer of these hormones, the body is less effective at burning calories.

A combination of increasing fat and loss of muscle generally leads to a change in body composition. Most new fat accumulates around the belly (intra-abdominal fat), which tends to be more inflammatory. This midlife middle, though common, isn't healthy.

Certainly, weight gain can be frustrating, especially if you're eating and exercising like you always have. Understand that this is a common occurrence and that you're not alone in your efforts to maintain or achieve a healthy weight. For women, a recent study suggests that perimenopause, the transition period before menopause, may be a good time to focus on lifestyle changes to improve metabolism and body composition.

The dangers of obesity

Feeling a little plump around the middle is common and can be one of the telltale signs of getting older. But too much weight can be dangerous to your health no matter what your age. Obesity is associated with several diseases:

- **Diabetes.** Excess fat makes your body resistant to insulin, the hormone that helps transport sugar (glucose) from your blood to individual cells, primarily muscle cells. When your body is resistant to insulin, your cells can't get the sugar they need for energy, resulting in diabetes. Obesity is a leading cause of type 2 diabetes. If you're at risk of developing diabetes, you may be able to avoid the disease by losing weight.

- **High blood pressure.** As fat cells accumulate, your body produces more blood to keep the new tissue supplied with oxygen and nutrients. More blood traveling through your arteries means added pressure on your artery walls. Weight gain also typically increases insulin. Increased insulin is associated with sodium and water retention, another contributor to increased blood volume. In addition, excess weight is often associated with increased heart rate and reduced capacity of blood vessels to transport blood. These two factors can increase your blood pressure and lead to a burst blood vessel.

- **High cholesterol.** The same dietary choices that lead to obesity often result in elevated levels of low-density lipoprotein (LDL, or "bad") cholesterol and reduced levels of high-density lipoprotein (HDL, or "good") cholesterol. Obesity is also associated with high triglycerides, another type of blood fat. Abnormal blood-fat levels can cause a buildup of fatty deposits (plaques) in your arteries, putting you at risk of heart attack and stroke.

- **Heart attack.** Excess weight can lead to fatty material building up in the vessels (arteries) that carry blood to your organs. If the coronary arteries that supply blood to your heart get damaged and clogged, a heart attack can result.

- **Osteoarthritis.** Obesity increases the risk of osteoarthritis due to increased wear and tear on joints. Chronic inflammation associated with obesity can also contribute to the development of the disease.

- **Sleep apnea.** Being overweight contributes to a large neck and narrowed airways, increasing the development of sleep apnea. Left untreated, sleep apnea can lead to a heart attack.

- **Cancer.** Several types of cancer are associated with being overweight. In women, these include breast, uterus, colon, and gallbladder cancers. Overweight men have a higher risk of colon and prostate cancers.

Responding to your risks

If your weight falls into the obese category, don't forget that losing just a few pounds can benefit your health. A modest reduction in weight — 3% to 10% of your total weight — can improve many conditions associated with excess weight.

The number you see when you step on the scale is in large part a product of your long-term habits. And just as your daily choices can lead you to gain weight over time, so too can your choices help you lose weight. You probably won't be able to lose the pounds you've put on all at once, but gradual changes over time produce healthier habits that can result in a slimmer you.

The changes outlined in Chapters 14 and 15 and other chapters in this book can collectively contribute to better health. If you focus on improving your habits in terms of diet, exercise, sleep and other behaviors, you should lose weight. Slow and steady weight loss of 1 or 2 pounds a week is considered the safest way to lose weight and the best way to keep it off.

We understand that weight loss isn't easy. If you need help, don't be afraid to ask for it. There are many medical professionals who can help you achieve a healthier weight, including registered dietitians, endocrinologists and gastrointestinal (GI) physicians who specialize in obesity. Start by talking with your primary health care provider, who can connect you with the appropriate individuals to assist you.

The rewards of a healthier weight are many. Not only will your health improve; you'll feel better physically. You'll have more energy for the things that you look forward to doing, such as travel, hobbies and spending time with your grandchildren. And you'll feel better about yourself. If you've been frustrated because of your weight, the boost in self-esteem from losing even a few pounds can be a welcome change.

SLEEP AND HEALTH

As busy as your days may be, sleep may seem like an afterthought. But sleep is a basic necessity, as fundamental to your health and well-being as fresh air and nutritious food. Sleep allows your body to take a break from its daytime operations. The renewal that sleep provides impacts your emotional reactions, physical energy, brain function, mental focus and even your immune system.

During sleep your body typically goes into energy conservation mode. Your muscles relax and your blood pressure drops about 10% to 15%. Brain activity quiets down during most stages of sleep. Oxygen consumption decreases approximately 10% and your body's core temperature drops.

At the same time, certain restorative activities increase during sleep. For example, brain systems perform a rapid clearing of potentially toxic waste products, such as the amyloid beta proteins that are closely linked to Alzheimer's disease. In addition, sleep allows time for cells to repair themselves and for new cells to develop.

Lack of sleep disrupts these key processes, and ongoing sleep deprivation impacts our long-term health. Sleep problems are linked to a number of chronic conditions, including cardiovascular disease, depression, high blood pressure and diabetes. Ultimately, this can affect your health span and life span.

Age and sleep

Sleep patterns tend to change with age. Most people find that as they get older, they have more difficulty falling asleep, and they wake up earlier in the morning. The transition to waking up may also become more abrupt, which may make you feel like you've become a lighter sleeper than when you were younger.

With age, you also tend to spend less time in deep, dreamless sleep. In addition, older adults often lose the ability to sleep in long stretches, called sleep continuity. You may awaken more often during the night — an average of three or four times each night. Health conditions that tend to become more prevalent with age, such as needing to go to the bathroom and feeling discomfort or pain from long-term (chronic) illnesses, may interrupt your sleep.

Among women, the transition into perimenopause and menopause can affect sleep. Nearly 40% of women report increased sleep challenges at this period in their lives. Hormonal changes and the symptoms associated with them, such as hot flashes, anxiety, and depression, frequently alter women's sleep patterns.

Many other factors can conspire to make it harder to get a good night's sleep as you get older. They include:

- **Lifestyle changes.** With age, you may become less physically or socially active. Activity helps promote good sleep. Individuals who have more free time on their hands may drink more caffeine or alcohol or take a daily nap. These things can interfere with nighttime sleep.
- **Medical conditions and life changes.** Chronic pain from conditions such as arthritis, fibromyalgia or back problems can disrupt sleep. Other illnesses that can interfere with sleep include acid reflux, dementia and lung disease. With age, men often develop noncan-

cerous enlargement of the prostate gland, called benign prostatic hyperplasia, or BPH. This can lead to more frequent urination at night. In women, hot flashes associated with menopause can disrupt sleep. If your partner snores, which tends to become more common with age, this can also affect your sleep.

- **Mental health issues.** Depression, stress and bereavement are common as people get older and cope with life changes such as physical limitations, loss of loved ones and leaving their homes. These conditions often cause sleep difficulties.
- **Medications.** Many medications have stimulating effects and can cause sleep difficulties. Medications that can interfere with sleep include some antidepressants, decongestants, bronchodilators, corticosteroids and some high blood pressure drugs. In addition, many over-the-counter sleep aids actually can be counterproductive to good sleep.
- **Sleep disorders.** Several sleep disorders become more common with age. These include sleep apnea, restless legs syndrome, periodic limb movement disorder and rapid eye movement (REM) sleep behavior disorder.

Despite all these factors, however, poor sleep isn't inevitable with age. There are

HOW MUCH SLEEP DO YOU NEED?

How much sleep each of us needs varies from person to person. In general, 7 to 8 hours of sleep is the amount that most people require to feel rested and is the amount associated with the lowest mortality risk. And contrary to popular opinion, you don't need less sleep as you get older. Adults require about the same amount of sleep from their 20s into old age.

If you don't feel rested on waking in the morning and you feel tired or sleepy during the day, it may be that you're not getting enough sleep, your sleep has become fragmented, you have a sleep disorder or your timing is off.

To help determine if you're getting enough sleep, a good tip is to try to wake up without an alarm clock. If you need an alarm to awaken, it's possible you may not be getting enough sleep.

many things you can do to improve the quality of your sleep.

How poor sleep influences health

Scientists have done a lot of research on what happens when we don't get enough sleep. Sleep deprivation can have a negative effect on practically every system and organ in our bodies.

Brain resources and memory

Sleep allows our brains time to heal and rejuvenate. When we don't get enough sleep, we tend to feel tired and blah. Our brain cells don't communicate as well and our concentration levels decrease, as does our ability to remember. Lack of sleep weakens our reaction times, shortens our attention spans and leaves us more prone to making mistakes. Even a single night of sleep deprivation can affect our ability to think logically, perform complex tasks and focus on multiple goals simultaneously.

Emotions and decision-making

Sleep disruption is frequently associated with depression, anxiety and burnout. Lack of sleep can lead to impulsive behav-

ior, poor judgment and irritability. As you go without sleep, your decision-making suffers. Interestingly, evidence shows that for every hour that you're awake during the day, the healthiness of the food you choose to eat decreases by 2%.

Immune system

As you read in Chapter 8, when you're tired, even from just one night of poor sleep, brain regulation of the immune system weakens, making you more susceptible to infections. Sleep helps our bodies fight off sickness and feel better. If you aren't sleeping like you should, you're more likely to develop an illness such as a cold or flu. Plus, if you do become ill, you can't fight sickness as effectively, and recovery takes longer.

Studies show that the relationship between sleep and the immune system is a two-way street. Activation of the immune system by an infection can disturb sleep, but it can also make you sleep longer and deeper, allowing your body to conserve energy for recovery.

Lack of quality sleep also produces cellular stress, which can lead to a mild yet chronic activation of the body's inflammatory response, as discussed in Chapter 1. Sleep offers the body's reparative processes a chance to decrease the daily damage from inflammation. Too little sleep makes for a double whammy — not only is your body unable to repair existing inflammatory damage, but more damage piles on.

Heart and blood vessels

A lot of evidence supports the importance of adequate rest for the health of your heart and blood vessels. Disrupted sleep leads to changes in blood pressure. High variability in how long you sleep or when you go to sleep is associated with higher blood pressure, abnormal cholesterol levels and insulin resistance.

Not getting enough sleep has been linked to an increased risk of heart attack. But getting just one additional hour of sleep a night can decrease that risk by 20%, according to some estimates. The link between lack of sleep and cardiovascular disease is likely caused by the chronic inflammation that poor sleep tends to promote.

Obesity and metabolism

Sleep loss can affect your metabolism by impairing your body's sensitivity to insulin and interfering with blood sugar function, which increases your risk of diabetes. Poor or restricted sleep can also impact hormones such as leptin and ghrelin, which affect your appetite. Ghrelin, when increased, makes you hungry, and lack of sleep will increase your ghrelin levels.

Disruption of these hormones' normal functions may lead you to eat more than you normally would when you're well rested. There's mounting evidence that people who get less than seven or eight hours of sleep a night have a higher risk of weight gain and obesity.

Skin

Studies suggest there may be a connection between sleep and the quality of your skin. One study found that people who slept between seven and nine hours a night had skin that was more moisturized and could protect and heal itself better after exposure to ultraviolet light than people who slept five hours a night or less. Skin quality, however, is affected by many other factors, including weight.

Responding to your risks

Understanding that a good night's sleep is key to sustaining your short- and long-term health, you should treat getting enough sleep with the same level of importance as taking a medication or daily vitamin.

Sleep is when the body rejuvenates, repairs and replenishes itself. When we don't allow that to happen properly, our bodies age quicker and we develop noncommunicable chronic diseases earlier in life. Like any medicine, sleep must be taken regularly. To make the most of your nightly dose of sleep, consider these important factors.

Make sleep a priority

Your bedtime schedule may be affected by all of the other events that fill your evenings. Relaxing after work, making dinner, fitting in loads of laundry and watching TV are all activities that may take place in the late afternoon and early evening and affect when you go to bed.

There's nothing wrong with these activities — they help close out the day and wrap up daily goals. All too often, though, these seemingly important events encroach on bedtime, narrowing the time allotted to sleep. If you're not careful, sleep ends up last on your list of priorities.

Set and follow a regular bedtime and waketime every day. It should be the same during the week as on the weekend. This may mean you need to tweak things here and there — start dinner a little earlier, divvy up tasks or limit TV viewing to one episode of a series instead of two or three — to achieve a reasonable bedtime.

Try not to spend more than eight hours in bed. If you have difficulty sleeping during the night, don't sleep in. Stick to your normal rising time and try to make up for the lost sleep the next night.

Develop bedtime rituals

Most of us need rituals to help us get ready for sleep. You might already have your own preferred bedtime routine. Maybe this involves prepping coffee for the morning, taking a warm bath, getting into comfortable pajamas, meditating or reading. If you need to establish a bedtime ritual, include activities that relax you and prepare you for sleep.

The goal is to signal to our brains that rest is imminent. Because brain activity is so integral to sleep, it's important to get the message through. We need to tell our brains that the day's labor is done and that outlying stressors and anxieties can be set aside until tomorrow. About an hour or so before you go to bed, start to slow down and begin your ritual. Doing so sends messages to your brain and the rest of your body that the restorative functions of sleep are about to take place.

Limit electronic devices

Not using electronic devices or watching TV for at least a half-hour before bed can help improve sleep quality. Watching TV or using your computer or other device too close to bedtime can be disruptive to your sleep because your mind stays engaged in what you just saw or heard rather than focused on falling asleep. There's some evidence that the blue light emitted by our phones can suppress melatonin, the hormone our brain produces in response to darkness.

Avoid naps

Your body only needs 7 to 8 hours of sleep a night, and napping during the day can interfere with better sleep at night. If you don't get a good night's sleep, the best strategy is to make up the lost sleep the following night rather than sleeping during the day. If you need to nap during the day, try to keep your nap to 20 minutes or less.

Exercise and stay active

Regular activity helps promote a good night's sleep. Aim for at least 150 minutes of moderate aerobic activity or 75 minutes of vigorous aerobic activity a week. Plan to exercise at least a few hours before bedtime. Exercise stimulates the brain and body, and exercising too close to bedtime may keep you awake.

Limit food and beverages before bed

Going to bed on a full stomach can make it harder to get a good night's sleep. Drinking alcohol or caffeine too close to bedtime can have the same effect. Alcohol, especially, promotes sleep onset, but sleep becomes much more fragmented, and you may have to get up to go to the bathroom. Too much water before bed can have the same effect.

Create a comfortable environment

Keep your sleeping environment quiet, dark and comfortably cool. Make sure your bed is comfortable.

Schedule worry time

If worries keep you awake, try to deal with them before bedtime. Set aside a worry time during the day. Make a list of problems and identify possible solutions.

Check your medications

If you continue to have difficulty sleeping, ask your health care provider if your medications may be contributing to your problem. Check over-the-counter

WHAT ABOUT SLEEP MEDICATIONS?

Sleeping pills may help in certain situations, such as when stress, travel or other disruptions keep you awake. If you regularly have trouble either falling or staying asleep — commonly known as insomnia — make an appointment to see your health care provider. The best way to manage the condition often depends on what's causing it. Identifying and managing an underlying cause, such as a medical condition or a sleep-related disorder, is a much more effective approach than just treating the symptom of insomnia itself.

Behavior changes learned through cognitive behavioral therapy are generally the best treatment for ongoing insomnia. Following a regular sleep schedule, exercising regularly, avoiding caffeine later in the day, avoiding daytime naps and keeping stress in check are also likely to help. But there are times when the addition of prescription sleeping pills may help you get some much-needed rest.

All prescription sleeping pills have risks, especially for people with certain medical conditions, including liver or kidney disease, and for older adults. Always talk with your health care provider before trying a new treatment for insomnia, even an over-the-counter product.

If you're going to reach for a sleep aid, natural melatonin is considered safe. Your brain produces this hormone in response to darkness. Taking a little extra may help to get your body's circadian rhythms in proper alignment.

products to see if they contain caffeine or other stimulants.

YOUR SKIN AND HAIR

Skin and hair changes are among the most visible signs of aging. Some of the first indications that you're getting older are changes to your skin, such as the development of fine lines and wrinkles. Everyone experiences skin changes at some point. How fast your skin ages is influenced by many factors, including heredity, nutrition, smoking, exposure to sunlight, your weight, quality of sleep and your sex life.

Your hair is another visible indication of the aging process. With time, hair starts to lose its color and turn gray. It may develop a different texture and become thinner. Many individuals, especially men, experience baldness in their later years.

Skin and aging

Skin is the body's largest organ. It protects against heat, sunlight, injury and infection. Skin helps control body temperature and stores water, fat and vitamin D. The skin has several layers, but the three main layers are the epidermis (top or outer layer), the dermis (middle layer) and the subcutis (lower or inner layer), where fat is stored.

Skin changes that occur with age are influenced by several changes in the body, including a decrease in production of the protein collagen, reduced blood flow, lower lipid levels and the loss of connective tissues just below the surface of the skin. Over time, these changes can cause your skin to become thinner, drier and less elastic.

One of the most visible indications of aging skin is the development of wrinkles. Over time, your skin naturally becomes less elastic and more thin. Decreased production of natural oils dries the skin and makes it appear more wrinkled. Fat in the deeper layers of your skin diminishes. This leads to loose, saggy skin and more pronounced lines and crevices.

Ultraviolet radiation, which speeds the natural aging process, is the primary cause of early wrinkling. Exposure to ultraviolet light breaks down your skin's connective tissues — collagen and elastin fibers, which lie in the deeper layer of skin called the dermis. This is why people who don't spend much time in the sun often look younger than their actual age. Smoking can accelerate the normal aging process of your skin, contributing to wrinkles. This may be due to tobacco's effect on collagen. And smoking causes your skin to take on a yellow and leathery appearance.

In addition to wrinkling, with age your skin becomes more prone to the development of lesions and blemishes. Exposure to sunlight destroys the ability of the skin to produce melatonin in certain areas, which is why your skin may develop white spots. The brown spots are where there's too much pigment.

Age spots, also known as liver spots, may begin to appear. These small, flat patches look like freckles. Skin lesions known as seborrheic keratoses (sometimes called barnacles) become more common with age. These are brown, black or light tan growths that are waxy or scaly in appearance and lightly raised. Other skin growths more commonly seen in older age include skin tags and angiomas, which are benign blood vessel growths.

Production of natural skin oils slows with age. The loss of oils can cause red, scaly and itchy skin on your back, legs, arms or elsewhere. Older individuals also tend to bruise more easily than younger people, and it can take longer for bruises to heal. Some medicines or illnesses may cause easier bruising.

Blue-eyed, fair-skinned people show more age-related skin changes. People of Black, Asian or Latino ancestry tend to have fewer wrinkles and smoother skin as they grow older. Yet people with skin of color have distinct concerns, such as changes in pigmentation and changes in facial structure. Older Black individuals typically exhibit increased skin thickness, contributing to reduced wrinkles but noticeable sagging of the skin below the chin or jawline (jowling). East Asian populations are predisposed to hyperpigmentation. Latino individuals' skin can also age differently.

Many skin conditions can be treated with lotions and creams that add moisture and relieve itching. But some skin conditions are more serious.

Skin cancer

Skin cancer — the abnormal growth of skin cells — most often develops on skin exposed to the sun. But this common form of cancer can also occur on areas of your skin not ordinarily exposed to sunlight. Skin cancer often begins in the epidermis, which is made up of three kinds of cells:

- **Squamous cells.** Thin, flat cells that form the top layer of the epidermis. Cancer that forms in squamous cells is called squamous cell carcinoma of the skin.
- **Basal cells.** Round cells under the squamous cells. Cancer that forms in basal cells is called basal cell carcinoma.
- **Melanocytes.** Found in the lower part of the epidermis, these cells make melanin, the pigment that gives skin its natural color. When skin is exposed to the sun, melanocytes make more pigment and cause the skin to tan or darken. Cancer that forms in melanocytes is called melanoma.

Melanoma is much less common than squamous and basal skin cancer but much more likely to invade nearby tissue and spread to other parts of the body. Most deaths from skin cancer are caused by melanoma.

While anyone of any skin color can get skin cancer, people with fair skin that freckles easily are the most susceptible. You can reduce your risk of skin cancer by limiting or avoiding exposure to ultraviolet (UV) radiation. Checking your skin for suspicious changes can help detect skin cancer at its earliest stages. Early detection of skin cancer gives you the greatest chance for successful skin cancer treatment.

Responding to your risks

You can't undo years of sun exposure, but you can protect your skin from further damage to slow the aging process and reduce the risk of skin cancer. An important principle is to do something small every day for your skin. Don't wait until problems pile on and then try to fix them.

Limit sun exposure

Sun protection is essential. You can protect your skin by seeking shade when outdoors and covering up with sun-protective clothing, such as a lightweight and long-sleeved shirt, pants, a wide-brimmed hat and sunglasses with ultraviolet protection. For more effective protection, look for clothing with an ultraviolet protection factor (UPF) label. If possible, try to avoid the sun between 10 a.m. and 2 p.m., when ultraviolet rays are strongest.

Wear a broad-spectrum sunscreen

If you're going to be outdoors, apply sunscreen to all skin that isn't covered by clothing, even in the winter. A broad-spectrum, water-resistant sunscreen with a sun protection factor (SPF) of 30 or higher provides good protection. The kind of sunscreen you use is a matter of personal choice. The best type is the one you will use again and again. If you have sensitive skin, opt for a sunscreen that contains titanium oxide and zinc oxide, which are known as physical blockers. Otherwise, you may want to try a sunscreen with chemicals such as oxybenzone, avobenzone, octisalate, octocrylene, homosalate and octinoxate. These formulations have a good texture and tend to rub into the skin without leaving a white film.

Apply sunscreen generously and reapply it every two hours — or more often if you're swimming or perspiring. Use a generous amount on all exposed skin, including your lips, the tips of your ears and the backs of your hands and neck.

Check your skin regularly

Examine your skin often for new skin growths or changes in existing moles, freckles, bumps and birthmarks. With the help of mirrors, check your face, neck, ears and scalp. Examine your chest, trunk and the tops and undersides of your arms and hands. Examine both the front and back of your legs and your feet, including the soles and the spaces between your toes. Check your genital area and between your buttocks. If you notice any changes, such as a mole that sticks out or looks different from other moles, let your health care provider know.

Stay away from tobacco

Smoking can speed up skin's normal aging process, contributing to wrinkles and other changes to the appearance of your face. These changes include crow's feet, pronounced lines between the eyebrows, an uneven skin complexion, a grayish tone on lighter skin, deep creases and puffiness below the eyes, wrinkles around the mouth and thinner lips.

Nicotine causes blood vessels to narrow, reducing the flow of oxygen and nutrients to the skin. Chemicals in tobacco smoke also trigger molecular events that alter or damage structures necessary for skin elasticity and health. Smoke that isn't inhaled may still dry and damage the surface of your skin.

Follow a skin-healthy diet

A healthy diet can help you look and feel your best. Eat plenty of fruits, vegetables, whole grains and lean proteins.

Protein is essential for healing and building new tissues, including skin tissue and hair. Without enough protein, skin becomes more fragile. Research suggests that a diet rich in fish oil or fish oil supplements and low in unhealthy fats and processed or refined carbohydrates might promote younger looking skin. Drinking plenty of water helps keep your skin hydrated.

Cleanse your skin gently

Perspiration, especially when wearing a hat or helmet or something tight against your skin, irritates the skin, so you want to wash your skin as soon as possible after sweating. Gently wash your skin to remove perspiration, pollution, makeup and other substances without irritating your skin. Scrubbing your skin clean can irritate your skin, and irritation may accelerate skin aging. After washing or bathing, gently pat or blot your skin dry with a towel so that some moisture remains on your skin.

Keep your skin moist

Moisturizers can't prevent wrinkles, but they can temporarily mask tiny lines and creases. To help relieve dryness and itching, take fewer baths and showers,

avoid strong soaps such as antibacterial soaps and increase the humidity in your home during the winter months.

Exercise regularly

A few studies suggest that moderate exercise improves circulation and boosts the body's immune system, in turn giving your skin a more youthful appearance.

Hair and aging

Hair color results from a pigment called melanin, which hair follicles produce. Hair follicles are structures in your skin that make and grow hair. Over time, the follicles make less melanin, and this causes hair to become gray. Graying often begins in your 30s, and the amount of graying you experience is largely determined by your genes. Gray hair tends to occur earlier in white individuals and later in people of Asian descent. Over-the-counter products can cover up the gray, but there isn't any product, including nutritional supplements or vitamins, that will stop or decrease the rate of graying.

Over time you may also notice a change in your hair thickness. Hair is made of

DO OVER-THE-COUNTER SKIN PRODUCTS WORK?

The answer to this common question is, it depends. People buy nonprescription wrinkle creams and lotions with the hope that these products can reduce wrinkles and prevent or reverse damage caused by the sun. Whether they have any beneficial effect depends on the products' ingredients and how long you use them. Because over-the-counter wrinkle creams aren't classified as drugs, they're not required to undergo scientific research to prove their effectiveness. If you're looking for a face-lift in a bottle, you probably won't find it in nonprescription wrinkle creams. The benefits of these products are usually minimal.

Moisturizing alone can improve the appearance of your skin. It temporarily plumps the skin, making lines and wrinkles less visible. Moisturizers are lotions, creams, gels and serums made of water, oils and other ingredients, such as proteins, waxes, glycerin, lactate and urea. Wrinkle creams are often moisturizers with active ingredients that offer additional benefits. The added ingredients are intended to improve skin tone and texture and reduce fine lines and wrinkles. The effectiveness of these products depends in part on your skin type and the active ingredients. The following are commonly found in skin products and may result in some improvement in the appearance of your skin.

- **Retinoids.** This term is used for vitamin A compounds, such as retinol and retinoic acid. These ingredients have long been used topically to help repair sun-damaged skin and reduce fine lines and wrinkles.
- **Vitamin C (ascorbic acid).** Vitamin C is a potent antioxidant, which means it protects the skin from free radicals — unstable oxygen molecules that break down skin cells and cause wrinkles. Vitamin C may help protect skin from sun damage and reduce fine lines and wrinkles. Before and between uses, wrinkle creams containing vitamin C must be stored so they are protected from air and sunlight.
- **Hydroxy acids.** Alpha hydroxy acids (AHAs) include glycolic, citric and lactic acid. They're used to remove dead skin cells (exfoliate). Using an AHA product regularly allows your skin to better absorb other products and stimulates the growth of smooth, evenly pigmented new skin. AHAs, beta hydroxyl acids and polyhydroxy acids have also been shown to be effective in reducing fine lines and wrinkles.

- **Coenzyme Q10.** This ingredient may help reduce fine wrinkles around the eyes and protect the skin from sun damage.
- **Peptides.** These molecules occur naturally in living organisms and are building blocks of proteins. Certain peptides may stimulate collagen production, improve skin texture and diminish wrinkling.
- **Tea extracts.** Green, black and oolong tea contain compounds with antioxidant and anti-inflammatory properties. Wrinkle creams are most likely to use green tea extracts.
- **Grape seed extract.** In addition to its antioxidant and anti-inflammatory properties, grape seed extract promotes collagen production.
- **Niacinamide.** A potent antioxidant, this substance is related to vitamin B-3 (niacin). It helps reduce water loss in the skin and may improve skin elasticity.

Because the Food and Drug Administration doesn't evaluate cosmetic products for effectiveness, there's no guarantee that any over-the-counter product will reduce wrinkles. Therefore, consider these points when considering use of a wrinkle cream:

- **Cost.** Cost has no relationship to effectiveness. A wrinkle cream that's more costly may not be more effective than a less costly product.
- **Lower doses.** Nonprescription wrinkle creams contain lower concentrations of active ingredients than do prescription creams. So the results, if any, are limited and usually short-lived.
- **Multiple ingredients.** A product with two or three active ingredients isn't necessarily more effective than a product with just one. Likewise, using several anti-wrinkle products at the same time may irritate your skin rather than benefit it.
- **Daily use.** You'll likely need to use a wrinkle cream once or twice a day for many weeks before noticing any improvement. And once you discontinue using the product, your skin is likely to return to its original appearance.
- **Side effects.** Some products may cause skin irritation, rashes, burning or redness. Be sure to read and follow instructions. It may help to select products that don't cause allergic reactions (hypoallergenic) or acne (noncomedogenic).
- **Individual differences.** Just because a friend swears by a product doesn't mean it will work for you. No one product works the same for everyone.

many protein strands. A single hair strand has a normal life of between two and seven years. When a strand falls out it is replaced with a new hair. As you get older, your replacement hair tends to be thinner and have less pigment. So don't be surprised if the thick, coarse hair you had as a young adult eventually becomes fine, lighter colored and thinner.

Nearly everyone experiences some hair loss with age. How much hair you have on your body and head and how much you lose as you get older is primarily determined by your genes. A decline in male and female sex hormones also plays a role.

Men are more likely to lose hair as they age. By age 60, most men are at least partly bald. Male-pattern baldness typically involves a receding hairline and hair loss on top of the head. A smaller number of women develop female-pattern baldness. More commonly, a woman's part may widen, or her hair may look and feel considerably thinner.

In women, hormone changes after menopause can cause facial hair to grow and become coarser. This most often happens to hair on the chin and around the lips. Men, meanwhile, may grow longer and coarser eyebrow, ear and nose hair.

YOUR SEXUAL HEALTH

A healthy sexual relationship can positively affect all aspects of your life, including your physical health, self-esteem, and the glow of your skin. Though movies and television might suggest that sex is only for younger adults, this isn't true. As mentioned earlier, the need for intimacy is ageless.

Sexuality is the way we experience and express ourselves sexually. It involves feelings, desires, and actions and can include different types of physical touch or stimulation. Intimacy is a feeling of closeness and connectedness in a relationship that can occur with or without a physical component.

It's a common misconception that women lose interest in having sex as they get older. While sexual activity tends to decline with age, some men and women continue to have vaginal intercourse, oral sex, and masturbate even in their 80s and 90s. Sexuality is driven by many factors, including your psychological health, physical health, the health of your relationship with your partner, and even societal taboos and expectations. It's important to understand the difference between age-related changes in sexual function and the effects of health changes on sexual function.

Common age-related changes

Aging brings life transitions that can create opportunities for older adults to redefine what sexuality and intimacy mean to them. Some older adults strive for both a sexual and intimate relationship, some are content with one without the other, and still others may choose to avoid these types of connections.

One of the more common sexual changes that occurs with age is a gradual slowing of physical response time. It takes longer to become aroused, to reach orgasm, and to be ready to have sex again.

For women, most physical and sexual changes are linked to menopause and reduced estrogen levels. The vagina can shorten and narrow and it takes longer for the vagina to swell and lubricate when you're sexually aroused. The vagina's walls also become thinner, drier and less elastic.

These changes can make intercourse less comfortable. After menopause, some women also experience waning levels of sexual interest. This actually has more to do with a decrease in the hormone testosterone than estrogen. Testosterone regulates your sex drive, whether you're a man or a woman.

As men age, they may find it takes longer to achieve an erection. Erections may be less firm, and some men may not ejaculate with orgasm. You may also need more time between ejaculations. Aging doesn't cause erectile dysfunction (impotence), but older men are more likely to have it. Common causes are alcohol abuse, medications, smoking, diabetes, atherosclerosis and side effects of prostate surgery.

Conditions that aren't typical

Since sexuality is so subjective and involves both physiological and psychological aspects, it's hard to define what's not typical. With this in mind, "not typical" is anything that makes sexual activity uncomfortable or that feels like a negative impact on the quality of your sex life.

Certain illnesses, disabilities, medicines and surgeries can affect your ability to have or enjoy sex. This includes conditions such as arthritis, chronic pain, dementia, depression, diabetes and incontinence. Stress is another leading cause of sexual difficulties.

Among women, surgeries such as mastectomy or hysterectomy can lead to a loss of sexual interest or the worry of being viewed as less desirable or less attractive. Among men, prostate gland surgery can result in erectile dysfunction or urinary incontinence, causing feelings of inadequacy.

Fortunately, there are treatments and therapies that can help in many of these situations — from medication to talk (cognitive) therapy. And remember that loss of interest in sex isn't always a

MENOPAUSE IS PART OF AGING

Years ago, conversations about perimenopause and menopause tended to be quieter. They might have occurred among your sisters or close friends, or they didn't happen at all. Often, the conversations were tinged with cultural taboos and some personal shame regarding changes in sexual function and desire. This was partly due to the fact that the medical establishment often treated menopause as a pathology — a condition or illness — rather than a natural part of aging.

Times are changing. Increasingly, women are speaking frankly with their health care providers about how to improve their sex lives as they experience symptoms of perimenopause and menopause. They want to continue to enjoy sexual intercourse and intimacy, despite the changes taking place with their reproductive health.

The good news is there are many options for managing the changes that come with menopause — from creams and lubricants to lifestyle changes — so that you can continue to enjoy a rewarding sex life.

For some women, menopause brings empowerment. They no longer have to worry about getting pregnant, their kids are grown and out of the house, and there's less need to guard their privacy. Because of this, their later years can mean more space for intimacy and sexual curiosity, even if extra care is required to make sex comfortable.

problem. Many people, both single individuals and couples, are perfectly happy with a decrease in their sex lives. You may find satisfaction in your relationships in other ways.

Nurturing a healthy sex life

Physical changes with age certainly don't mean that your sex life is over, but you may have to redefine some of your expectations and assumptions. A healthy sex life depends on your mental state as much as your physical health. If you're embarrassed or ashamed of your changing sexual needs, anxiety can get the best of you and interfere with your ability to become aroused. The stress of worrying too much about performance can trigger impotence in men or a lack of arousal in women. If you're having sexual difficulties, a good first step is to talk with your health care provider.

A healthy sex life often is linked to good communication with your partner. Ask questions: Are we having fun? What do you like and what's uncomfortable? Do you want to do things differently? What helps you to get in the mood?

Often, simple changes can improve your sex life. You might change the time of day when you have sex to a time when you have more energy. Because it may take longer to become aroused, take time to set the stage for romance, such as a candlelight dinner or an evening of dancing. Or you might try a new sexual position.

You might also consider talking to a therapist who can help you with some of your emotional hurdles and offer strategies to improve intimacy in your relationships, all of which will help improve your sex life.

Finally, taking good care of your overall health — physical as well as mental — will benefit your sex life. This includes eating a healthy diet, enjoying regular exercise, getting enough sleep and reducing stress. You might also want to avoid or limit alcohol, as excessive alcohol decreases sexual function in both men and women. Plus, a healthy diet and regular exercise can help you to keep your weight in check. There's a connection between weight and sex. Studies have found that overweight men who lose weight generally have improved sexual experiences, as well as improved erectile function and reduced risk of erectile dysfunction.

Additional steps that may help improve sexual satisfaction among women include the following:

Use lubricant

Dyspareunia, defined as difficult or painful intercourse, and vaginal dryness are common problems in 80% of post-menopausal women. If you're experiencing vaginal dryness, try a vaginal moisturizer or lubricant. Regular intercourse helps to maintain lubrication and keeps genital tissues more supple.

Consider hormone therapy

If over-the-counter products aren't helpful, talk to your health care provider about estrogen therapy. Estrogen therapy is an effective treatment option for relieving menopausal symptoms. Depending on your personal and family medical history, your doctor may recommend estrogen in the lowest dose and for the shortest time frame needed to provide symptom relief for you. If you still have your uterus, you'll need progestin in addition to estrogen.

Long-term use of hormone therapy may have some cardiovascular and breast cancer risks, but starting hormones around the time of menopause has shown benefits for some women. Talk to your doctor about the benefits and risks of hormone therapy and whether it's a safe choice for you.

WHAT DO YOU THINK?

As you reflect on what you just read and contemplate your future health, ask yourself these questions.

- *How do I feel about my current well-being?*
- *What am I doing now that I feel good about?*
- *What are some aspects of my general well-being I'd like to improve?*
- *What changes can I make that I'm most likely to stick with?*

A recent position paper from the North American Menopause Society suggests that hormone therapy is helpful and safe for women younger than age 60 or within 10 years of menopause to improve bothersome symptoms and prevent bone loss. For women who are more than 10 years from menopause, the risks of heart disease, stroke, vein blood clots and dementia start to outweigh the benefits.

Hormone therapy may also help relieve discomfort with intercourse and some urinary symptoms.

10

Cancer

Aging is the most important risk factor for the development of cancer. The vast majority of cancers are diagnosed in individuals age 50 and older. While there's no surefire way to prevent cancer, you can reduce your risk by making healthy choices throughout your life, including keeping up to date with recommended screening tests.

Why cancer develops in some people but not in others isn't fully known. But as medical professionals continue to gain knowledge about what may contribute to cancer development, we're learning more about possible ways to prevent it.

Your risk of cancer includes some factors that you can't control, such as your genes and your age. But there are a number of factors that you do have

influence over, including your lifestyle habits.

What can you do to reduce your cancer risk? Just under 30% of cancer deaths today are associated with smoking. Evidence suggests that another third of cancers may be related to dietary factors. Obesity plays a major role in cancer development. If Americans applied everything that's known about cancer prevention to their daily lives, cancer rates might be reduced significantly.

WHAT IS CANCER?

There are at least 200 different kinds of cancer. Some cancers affect just one organ, while others spread to nearby tissues or to other areas of the body. But the basic characteristic of all cancers is the same — uncontrolled growth and risk for potential spread of abnormal (malignant) cells.

Normally, human cells grow and divide in an orderly fashion. But sometimes the process runs amok — cells continue dividing without restraint, crowding out neighboring normal cells. This happens because cancer cells either lack the controls that switch off growth or they lose their ability to undergo natural death. As cancer cells increase in number, they compete with normal cells for essential nutrients and space, affecting normal cell functioning.

Why cancer develops is a basic question that scientists are still attempting to unravel, and it's likely that the answer may not always be the same. Researchers have yet to understand many of the exact processes by which cancer cells develop, grow, divide and communicate, but

they're learning a lot about what goes on within a cell that may cause it to turn cancerous. This knowledge is aiding the development of new treatments.

It's understandable that you may fear cancer, but know that no matter your age, it's never too late to set a course that could help you avoid cancer. This chapter contains information on the most common cancers — breast, lung, prostate and colorectal cancer — but be aware there are opportunities to modify, lower or prevent your risk for other cancers.

BREAST CANCER

The National Cancer Institute estimates about 1 in 8 women in the United States will develop breast cancer at some point during her lifetime. Risk of breast cancer increases with age, with most breast cancers occurring in women older than age 50. The median age at diagnosis is 63.

Breast cancer most commonly develops in breast ducts, small tubes designed to carry milk from the tiny sacs that produce milk (lobules) to the nipple. But cancer may also occur in the lobules or in other breast tissue.

The most common sign of breast cancer is a lump or thickening in the breast.

Often, the lump is painless. Other signs of breast cancer include:

- Spontaneous clear or bloody discharge from your nipple.
- A change in in the appearance of a nipple, or an inverted nipple, if it isn't normally inverted.
- A change in the size or contours of your breast.
- Any dimpling or puckering of the skin over your breast.
- Redness or pitting, and possible thickening, of the skin over your breast that makes it look similar to the skin of an orange.

Keep in mind that many breast changes aren't cancerous; still, it's important to see your health care provider if you notice anything unusual. Your provider may order a diagnostic mammogram to evaluate a breast concern. When breast cancer is detected and treated early — while the tumor is small and before cancerous cells have spread to neighboring tissues — the odds of successful treatment are very good.

Risk factors

Scientists don't know what causes most breast cancers. However, they do know that certain factors may increase your risk:

- **Sex.** Although men can develop breast cancer, it's primarily a disease of women. Only about 1 of every 100 cases occurs in men.
- **Age.** Your risk of breast cancer increases as you get older.
- **Personal history.** Having cancer in one breast increases your chances of developing it in the other. Your risk of breast cancer is also higher if you've had a breast biopsy that found lobular carcinoma in situ (LCIS) or atypical hyperplasia.
- **Family history.** Women who have a mother or sister diagnosed with breast cancer before age 50 have a greater chance of developing breast cancer themselves.
- **Genetic predisposition.** Defects in one of several genes, such as BRCA1 or BRCA2, put you at greater risk of developing breast cancer.
- **Excess weight.** Obesity increases breast cancer risk, especially after menopause.
- **Exposure to estrogen.** If you reach menopause late (after age 55) or begin menstruating before age 12, you have a higher risk of developing breast cancer. The same is true if you've never given birth or if your first pregnancy occurred after age 30.
- **Hormone therapy.** Women who take hormone therapy medications containing estrogen and progesterone for

more than 3 to 5 years to treat signs and symptoms of menopause have an increased risk of breast cancer. Risk of breast cancer decreases when women stop taking the medications.

- **Race.** White women are more likely to develop breast cancer than women of Black or Latino ancestry.

- **Exposure to radiation.** If you received substantial radiation treatments to your chest as a child or young adult, your risk of breast cancer is increased.

- **Alcohol use.** Drinking alcohol increases the risk of breast cancer. Data from the Women's Health Study found that women who drank between three and

BREAST CANCER SCREENING

Mammograms are commonly used to screen for breast cancer. A mammogram is an X-ray of the breast that can identify masses too small to be felt.

For women at average risk of breast cancer, doctors generally recommend screening mammograms beginning at age 40. If you're at high risk, screening may begin earlier. Exactly when to begin mammogram screening and whether to repeat it every year or every other year are decisions best discussed with your health care provider.

Also discuss with your provider whether you might benefit from additional screening. Some women have dense breasts — breasts with more ducts and glands than fat. This is common, but it increases the chance that breast cancer may go undetected on a mammogram because dense breast tissue can mask a potential tumor. There's some evidence that supplemental tests, such as a 3D mammogram or breast MRI, may be more effective in detecting breast cancer in dense tissue.

Make sure to review the benefits, as well as risks and limitations, of supplemental tests with your health care provider and decide together what's best in your particular situation.

six glasses of wine a week were 15% more likely to develop breast cancer than were nondrinkers.

- **Smoking.** Some studies suggest that smoking may increase breast cancer risk.

LUNG CANCER

Lung cancer is the leading cause of cancer deaths in the United States among both men and women. Each year, it claims more lives than prostate, breast and colon cancers combined. The good news is that most lung cancer deaths are highly preventable. That's because smoking accounts for approximately 80% to 90% of lung cancers. But lung cancer also occurs in people who never smoked and in those who never had prolonged exposure to secondhand smoke. In these cases, there may be no clear cause of the cancer.

Lung cancer usually doesn't produce signs or symptoms until the disease is advanced. When symptoms do appear, they may include:

- Coughing — either a dry cough or one that produces sputum, which may contain blood.
- Shortness of breath.
- Chest pain.
- Hoarseness.
- Losing weight without trying.
- Fever.

If you experience any of these symptoms, see your health care provider. The earlier you discover and treat lung cancer, the better chance you have of lengthening your life.

Risk factors

Smoking is the greatest risk factor for lung cancer. Your risk increases with the number of cigarettes you smoke each day and the number of years you've smoked. Your risk is also greater if you start smoking early in life. Other known risk factors for lung cancer include:

- **Exposure to secondhand smoke.** Daily exposure to secondhand smoke may increase your chances of developing lung cancer by as much as 30%.
- **Exposure to radon gas.** Radon comes from the natural (radioactive) breakdown of uranium in soil, rock and water and eventually becomes part of the air you breathe. Unsafe levels can accumulate in buildings.
- **Exposure to other carcinogens.** Workplace exposure to cancer-causing substances such as asbestos, vinyl chloride, nickel chromates and coal products can increase your risk of lung cancer, especially if you're a smoker.

- **Previous radiation therapy.** If you've undergone radiation therapy to the chest for any other type of cancer, you may have an increased risk of developing lung cancer.
- **Family history.** People with a parent, sibling or child with lung cancer may have an increased risk of the disease.
- **Sex.** Women — current or former smokers — are at greater risk of lung cancer than are men who've smoked an equal amount. It's possible women may be more susceptible to cancer-causing substances found in tobacco or that the hormone estrogen plays a role.
- **Race.** Black men are slightly more likely to develop lung cancer than are white men. They also develop the disease at an earlier age.

PROSTATE CANCER

Prostate cancer is the most diagnosed cancer in men in the United States, aside from certain skin cancers, which are typically less life-threatening. The cancer develops in the prostate gland — the small, walnut-shaped gland that surrounds the bottom portion of a man's bladder and about the first inch of the urinary channel (urethra).

Approximately 1 in 8 men will be diagnosed with prostate cancer in his lifetime. As you age, your risk of prostate cancer increases. It's estimated that by age 50, about one-third of men have some cancerous cells in their prostate glands. By age 80, this increases to about three-quarters of all men.

Typically, prostate cancer grows slowly and remains confined to the prostate gland, where it usually doesn't cause serious harm. But not all prostate cancers act the same; some forms are aggressive and can spread quickly.

LUNG CANCER SCREENING

If you're at high risk of lung cancer because of your smoking history or exposure to harmful substances, you may want to consider low-dose computed tomography (CT) screening to look for early indications of possible disease.

Yearly screening is recommended for adults ages 50 to 80 with a 20-pack-a-year smoking history who still smoke or who quit within the past 15 years. Talk to your health care provider about whether you should be screened.

Prostate cancer often doesn't produce any symptoms in its early stages. That's why many cases aren't detected until they've spread beyond the gland. When signs and symptoms do occur, they may include:

- Sudden urge to urinate.
- Difficulty starting urination, as well as difficulty stopping urination.
- Pain during urination.
- Weak urine flow and dribbling.
- Intermittent urine flow.
- Sensation the bladder isn't empty after urination and needs to void again soon.
- Frequent urination at night.
- Blood in urine.
- Painful ejaculation.
- Dull pain in the lower pelvic area.
- General pain in the lower back, abdomen, hips and upper thighs.

Risk factors

There's no simple formula that predicts who will encounter prostate cancer and at what point in life. However, various factors — some of which you can control — affect your odds of developing prostate cancer. Research suggests that a combination of factors may play a role in prostate cancer risk:

- **Age.** As you get older, your risk of prostate cancer increases. It's most common after age 50.

- **Race.** For reasons not well understood, Black men have a greater risk of prostate cancer than do men of other races. They're also more likely to get prostate cancer at a younger age and to have an aggressive form.
- **Family history.** If your father or brother was diagnosed with prostate cancer, your risk of developing the disease is at least twice that of the average American male. Also, if you have a family history of genes that increase risk of breast cancer (BRCA1 or BRCA2) or a very strong family history of breast cancer, your risk of prostate cancer may be higher.
- **Obesity.** Individuals who are obese may have a higher risk of prostate cancer compared with those at a healthy weight, though studies have had mixed results.
- **Diet.** There's some evidence that a diet high in saturated and trans fats may increase your risk of prostate cancer and more advanced disease. The reason behind this isn't clear, though at least one study has hypothesized that high-fat diets may mimic the effects of cancer-causing genes. Other studies suggest that diets high in total calories and high in calcium and dairy products may increase the risk of prostate cancer. More research is needed.
- **Sexual activity.** The impact of sexual activity on prostate cancer risk is

controversial. Some past research suggested that men with a history of sexually transmitted infections (STIs) may be at higher risk of prostate cancer. However, a definitive relationship hasn't been proved and more research is needed. A recent study suggests that certain factors, such as fewer sexual partners over the course of a lifetime, may be associated with a lower prostate cancer risk.

- **Supplemental hormones.** Large doses of the nutritional supplement dehy-droepiandrosterone (DHEA) may increase prostate cancer risk.

COLORECTAL CANCER

Colon cancer begins in the large intestine (colon), the final part of the digestive tract. Colon cancer typically affects older adults, though it can happen at any age. It usually begins as small, noncancerous (benign) clumps of cells called polyps that form on the inside of the

PROSTATE CANCER SCREENING

A digital rectal exam and a blood test called the prostate-specific antigen (PSA) test may be used to screen for prostate cancer. The PSA test isn't foolproof, but it can identify an increase in a chemical compound produced in the prostate gland that's sometimes associated with prostate cancer.

If you're a man older than age 50 and you haven't been screened for prostate cancer, talk with your health care provider about whether screening is right for you. Also discuss the possible options if your PSA result comes back above normal. If you're Black or have a family history of prostate cancer, you may want to have this discussion earlier.

PSA screening is controversial. Though it can catch problems in their early stages, it can also give false-positive results that lead to other, unnecessary tests. A false positive is a test result that states that a condition or attribute is present when it's not.

COLORECTAL CANCER SCREENING

Most medical organizations recommend you begin screening around age 45. If you're at increased risk, your health care provider may recommend you start earlier. Different tests are used to screen for the disease. The one that's best for you depends on several factors, including your cancer risk, your personal preference and what's available.

- **Colonoscopy.** A flexible tube (colonoscope) is inserted into the rectum and threaded through the colon. A tiny video camera at the tip of the tube allows a doctor to detect changes or abnormalities inside the colon. It's one of the most sensitive tests currently available for colon cancer screening. The test requires a cleansing of the colon beforehand and sedation during the test.
- **Stool DNA.** This test uses a sample of your stool to look for DNA changes that may indicate cancer or precancerous conditions. It also checks for blood in your stool. You collect a stool sample at home and send it to a laboratory for testing. The test doesn't require bowel preparation or sedation, but it's less sensitive at detecting precancerous polyps than a colonoscopy.
- **Fecal occult blood test or fecal immunochemical test.** These tests check stool samples for hidden (occult) blood. Similar to a stool DNA test, stool collection can be performed at home. The tests aren't as sensitive as colonoscopy.
- **Virtual colonoscopy (CT colonography).** This test involves a CT scan of the colon and rectum to check for abnormalities. Unlike traditional colonoscopy, the test doesn't require sedation or the insertion of a scope into the colon. But it does require bowel cleansing beforehand, and it might not detect small polyps and cancers.
- **Flexible sigmoidoscopy.** A flexible tube is inserted into the rectum and lower third of the colon. A tiny video camera at the tip of the tube allows a doctor to detect changes or abnormalities. A major drawback of this test is that it doesn't examine the entire colon and some potentially cancerous lesions may be missed.

With some tests — stool DNA, fecal occult blood and fecal immunochemical tests and virtual colonoscopy — a follow-up colonoscopy may be necessary if an abnormality is detected because tissue samples can't be taken during the tests.

colon. Over time, some of these polyps can turn cancerous. Rectal cancer develops in the rectum, the last several inches of the colon.

Together, the two cancers are referred to as colorectal cancer. Colorectal cancer is one of the most common cancers diagnosed in men and women in the United States.

Doctors aren't certain what causes most colorectal cancers. Only a small percentage are linked to genes that you inherit. The cancer often doesn't produce any symptoms in its early stages. When symptoms do develop, they may include:

- A persistent change in your bowel habits, including diarrhea or constipation or a change in the consistency of your stool.
- Rectal bleeding or blood in your stool.
- Persistent abdominal discomfort, such as cramps, gas or pain.
- A feeling that your bowel doesn't empty completely.
- Weakness or fatigue.
- Unexplained weight loss.

Risk factors

There are several possible risk factors for developing colorectal cancer. Your lifestyle, diet, health conditions and family history can all play a role. Factors that may increase your risk of colorectal cancer include:

- **Age.** Colon cancer can be diagnosed at any age, but a majority of people with colon cancer are older than age 50. Rates of colon cancer in people younger than 50, however, have been increasing and doctors aren't sure why.
- **Race.** Black Americans of African ancestry have a greater risk of colon cancer than do people of other races. They also tend to develop colorectal cancer at an earlier age.
- **A personal history of colorectal cancer or polyps.** If you've already had colon cancer or noncancerous colon polyps, you have a greater risk of colon cancer in the future.
- **Inflammatory intestinal diseases.** Chronic inflammatory diseases of the colon, such as ulcerative colitis and Crohn's disease, can increase your risk of colon cancer.
- **Inherited syndromes.** Some genetic mutations passed on within families can significantly increase risk of colorectal cancer. The most common inherited syndromes that increase colon cancer risk are familial adenomatous polyposis (FAP) and Lynch syndrome, which is also known as hereditary nonpolyposis colorectal cancer (HNPCC). People with untreat-

ed FAP have a significantly increased risk of developing colorectal cancer before age 40.

- **Family history of colon cancer.** You're more likely to develop colon cancer if you have a blood relative who's had the disease. If more than one family member has had colon cancer or rectal cancer, your risk is even greater.
- **Low-fiber, high-fat diet.** Colorectal cancer may be associated with a diet low in fiber and high in fat and calories. Some studies suggest an increased risk of colon cancer in people whose diets are high in red meat and processed meat.
- **A sedentary lifestyle.** People who are inactive are more likely to develop colon cancer. Getting regular physical activity may reduce this risk.
- **Diabetes.** Individuals with diabetes or insulin resistance have an increased risk of colon cancer.
- **Obesity.** People who are significantly overweight have an increased risk of colon cancer and an increased risk of dying of colon cancer compared with individuals at a healthy weight.
- **Smoking and alcohol.** Individuals who smoke or consume large amounts of alcohol are at greater cancer risk.
- **Radiation therapy.** Radiation therapy that's directed at the abdomen to treat previous cancers can increase the risk of colon cancer.

REDUCING YOUR CANCER RISK

Scientists and researchers continue to gain ground in their quest to better understand how and why cancer occurs, so that one day all cancers can be successfully treated and perhaps even prevented. In the meantime, there's plenty that you can do to decrease your cancer risk. Cancer prevention often boils down to making a few key decisions in your everyday life. And understand that no matter your age, it's never too late to set a course that could help you avoid this common disease.

Don't smoke or use tobacco

Avoid tobacco and products such as marijuana. Research shows that smoking anything puts you on a collision course with cancer. Smoking has been linked to various types of cancer, including cancer of the lung, mouth, throat, larynx, pancreas, bladder, cervix and kidney. Chewing tobacco has been linked to cancer of the oral cavity and pancreas.

If you smoke, find a way to quit. Quitting now can significantly reduce your cancer risk — even if you've smoked for years. The benefits of stopping smoking begin immediately, and over the years, your odds of developing several types of cancer, especially lung cancer, decrease substantially.

If you need help quitting tobacco, ask your health care provider about stop-smoking products and other strategies for quitting. A combination of medication and behavioral therapy is often the most effective strategy for stopping smoking. Medications include nicotine replacement therapy as well as non-nicotine medications (Chantix, Zyban). Taking one or more of these drugs can increase your chances of being successful. Because use of the medications can be complicated, don't be afraid to ask your health care provider for a referral to a certified nicotine dependence counselor if one is available.

Even if you don't use tobacco personally, breathing in secondhand smoke can increase your risk of lung cancer. Take steps to protect yourself from exposure to secondhand smoke by avoiding areas where people may smoke.

Eat a healthy, balanced diet

Making good food selections at the grocery store and preparing healthy meals can't guarantee that you won't develop cancer, but these steps can have a significant impact on your risk.

Choose fruits, vegetables and other plant-based foods

These foods contain essential vitamins, minerals and antioxidants, which may help protect you from cancer. Antioxidants — found mainly in fruits and vegetables that are red, purple, blue and orange — are thought to improve nutrition and defend the body's cells from unstable and harmful molecules known as free radicals.

Damage to cells caused by free radicals, especially damage to DNA, may play a role in the development of cancer and other health conditions. Additional sources of antioxidants are nuts and grains, poultry and fish.

In addition to antioxidants, fruits and vegetables contain other chemical compounds that may be cancer protective. For example, certain compounds in cruciferous vegetables, such as broccoli, cabbage and bok choy, may be especially protective against lung cancer, while those in soy products may help protect against prostate and breast cancers.

Studies suggest that individuals who follow plant-based diets, such as the Mediterranean diet, appear to have a reduced risk of several cancers, including colorectal, breast, stomach, pancreas, prostate and lung cancers. A Mediterranean diet focuses mostly on plant-based foods, such as fruits and vegetables, whole grains, legumes and nuts. It also includes healthy fats, such as olive oil, and it advocates fish instead of red meat.

Limit sugar and fat

A diet high in sugar and unhealthy fats can contribute to an unhealthy eating pattern, resulting in excess body fat. Obesity places you at greater risk of several cancers, including breast and prostate cancers. To reduce your cancer risk and prevent obesity, try to eat lighter and leaner by limiting or avoiding high-calorie foods made from refined sugar and saturated and trans fats.

Limit processed meats

A report from the International Agency for Research on Cancer, the cancer agency of the World Health Organization, concluded that eating large amounts of processed meat can slightly increase the risk of certain cancers. Any meat that's been preserved by smoking, curing or salting is processed. Meats with added chemical preservatives are also processed.

See Chapter 15 for more on healthy eating.

Keep physically active

Exercise provides many beneficial effects, which are thought to play a role in reducing your risk of several cancers. Regular exercise:
• Prevents obesity.
• Strengthens the immune system.
• Improves circulation.
• Speeds digestion.
• Reduces inflammation.
• Lowers levels of sex hormones and growth factors associated with cancer development and progression.
• Prevents high levels of insulin, linked to cancer development and progression.
• Alters the metabolism of bile acids, decreasing exposure to the suspected carcinogens.

Any amount of physical activity provides some health benefits. As a general goal, include at least 30 minutes of physical activity in your daily routine, but be aware that more activity is even better. To reap greater health benefits, aim for at least 150 minutes a week of moderate aerobic activity or 75 minutes a week of vigorous aerobic activity. You can also do a combination of moderate and vigorous activity.

See Chapter 14 for information on developing an exercise program.

Maintain a healthy weight

As mentioned previously, a healthy weight can help reduce your risk of several cancers, including those of the breast, prostate, lung, colon and kidney. A balanced diet and regular exercise are often the best tools for losing weight. If your weight is currently healthy, try to maintain that weight as you get older, when people naturally tend to add on pounds.

See Chapter 9 for more information on weight and health.

Limit alcohol

If you drink alcohol, do so in moderation. The risk of various cancers — including cancer of the breast, colon, lung, kidney and liver — increases with the amount of alcohol you drink and the length of time you've been consuming alcohol regularly. If you drink alcohol, limit the amount. Moderate alcohol use for healthy adults generally means no more than one drink a day for women and no more than two drinks a day for men.

Protect yourself from the sun

Skin cancer is one of the most common kinds of cancer — and one of the most preventable. To reduce your risk, follow these tips:

- **Avoid the midday sun.** Stay out of the sun between 10 a.m. and 4 p.m., when the sun's rays are strongest.
- **Stay in the shade.** When you're outdoors, keep to the shade as much as possible. Sunglasses and a broad-brimmed hat help, too.
- **Cover exposed areas.** Wear tightly woven, loose-fitting clothing that covers as much of your skin as possible. Opt for dark colors, which absorb more ultraviolet radiation, keeping it from getting to your skin, than do white and pastel colors.
- **Don't skimp on sunscreen.** Use a broad-spectrum sunscreen with an SPF of at least 30, even on cloudy days. Apply sunscreen generously and reapply it every two hours — more often if you're swimming or perspiring.
- **Avoid tanning beds and sunlamps.** These are just as damaging as natural sunlight.

Get vaccinated

Cancer prevention includes protection from certain viral infections. Talk to your health care provider about vaccinations to help prevent the following infections:

- **Hepatitis B.** Hepatitis B can increase the risk of developing liver cancer. The hepatitis B vaccine is recommended for certain adults at high risk, such as those who are sexually active but not in a mutually monogamous relationship, people with sexually transmitted infections, people who use intravenous drugs, men who have unprotected sex with men, and health care or public safety workers who might be exposed to infected blood or body fluids.

- **Human papillomavirus (HPV).** HPV is a sexually transmitted virus that can lead to cervical and other genital cancers as well as squamous cell cancers of the head and neck. The HPV vaccine is recommended for girls and boys ages 11 and 12. The vaccine also is recommended for everyone through age 26, if they're not already vaccinated. Recently, the U.S. Food and Drug Administration approved the use of the vaccine Gardasil 9 for individuals up to age 45, but vaccination isn't recommended for everyone older than age 26.

Talk with your health care provider about these vaccinations, whether they're for you and your options.

Avoid risky behaviors

Another effective cancer prevention tactic is to avoid behaviors that can lead to infections which, in turn, might increase your cancer risk. For example:

- **Practice safe sex.** Limit your number of sexual partners and use a condom when you have sex. The more sexual partners you have in your lifetime, the more likely you are to contract a sexually transmitted infection such as HIV or HPV. People who have HIV or AIDS have a higher risk of cancer of the anus, liver and lung. HPV is most often associated with cervical cancer, but it might also increase the risk of cancer of the anus, penis, throat, vulva and vagina.

- **Don't share needles.** Sharing needles with people who use intravenous drugs can lead to HIV, as well as hepatitis B and hepatitis C, which can increase the risk of liver cancer. If you're concerned about drug misuse or addiction, seek professional help.

See your provider regularly

Regular self-exams and screenings for various types of cancers — such as skin, colon, cervix, breast and prostate — can increase your chances of discovering cancer early, when treatment is most likely to be successful. Ask your health care provider about the best cancer screening schedule for you.

For more information on recommended screenings, see Chapter 17.

Additional strategies

The following measures may influence risk of specific cancers.

Breast cancer

Additional steps that can help prevent breast cancer include:

- **Breastfeeding.** Breastfeeding may play a role in breast cancer prevention. The longer you breastfeed, the greater the protective effect. Some studies show that every 12 months of breastfeeding reduces the risk of breast cancer by about 4%.
- **Avoidance of hormone therapy.** Combination hormone therapy taken to help alleviate symptoms of menopause may increase the risk of breast cancer. Talk with your health care provider about the benefits and risks of this therapy. You may be able to manage your menopausal symptoms with exercise, dietary changes or nonhormonal therapies. If you decide

that the benefits of short-term hormone therapy outweigh the risks, use the lowest dose that works for you and have your provider monitor the length of time you're taking hormones.

- **Preventive medication.** If you're at high risk of breast cancer, you may be able to improve your odds of staying cancer-free with an approach known as preventive medication or risk reduction therapy. Medications used for breast cancer risk reduction include estrogen blockers, such as tamoxifen and raloxifene, and aromatase inhibitors, such as exemestane, which reduce the synthesis of estrogen in fatty tissue. They're generally taken daily for five years, but they're not without risks. The medications can produce side effects, including hot flashes or night sweats. Other risks include osteoporosis, uterine cancer and blood clots. It's important to discuss both the benefits and the risks of these medications with your doctor.

Lung cancer

To reduce your risk of lung cancer, also:

- **Pay attention to radon.** Check the levels in your home, especially in the basement. This is particularly important if you live in an area where radon is a known problem. The best tests are those that take between three and six months.

- **Be aware of toxic chemicals.** Take precautions to protect yourself from cancer-causing substances such as vinyl chloride, nickel chromates and coal products. Wear a face mask at work for protection and be certain that it fits correctly.

Colorectal cancer

Some medications may reduce your risk of developing precancerous polyps or colon cancer. For instance, there's evidence suggesting that regular use of aspirin or aspirin-like drugs may help deter the development of polyps and colon cancer. But it's not clear what dose and what length of time are needed to be of benefit, and taking aspirin daily has some risks, including gastrointestinal bleeding and ulcers.

Preventive medications are generally reserved for people at high risk of colon cancer. If you're at increased risk, discuss your risk factors with your health care provider to determine whether such medications are right for you.

WHAT DO YOU THINK?

As you reflect on what you just read and contemplate your future health, ask yourself these questions.

- *How do I feel about my current cancer risk?*
- *What am I doing now that I feel good about?*
- *What are some risk factors for cancer I'd like to improve?*
- *What changes can I make that I'm most likely to stick with?*

11

Frailty and recovery from injury

When you hear the term *frail* you may picture someone who's older, thin and hunched over. Frailty actually encompasses a larger group of individuals who may not "appear" frail but are at increased risk of poor health outcomes due to diverse health challenges.

Several studies show that an estimated 4% to 16% of Americans age 65 and older are frail. Individuals with pre-frailty — who fulfill some, but not all, criteria for frailty — range from 28% to 44%. While frailty becomes more common with age, it isn't synonymous with aging; not all people who live into their 70s and 80s and beyond are, or will become, frail.

Frailty is, however, a legitimate concern. It's associated with an increased risk of

infection and falls, a lower quality of life, a higher risk of hospitalization and skilled nursing facility admission, and an increased risk of death. Individuals who are frail are more likely to experience delayed recovery times and poorer outcomes when faced with any physical stress or challenge, such as surgery or a new disease.

The good news is that frailty can often be prevented or treated. Your efforts to live healthier and age well may help reduce your risk of becoming medically frail.

FRAILTY AND AGING

Among doctors and other members of the medical community, frailty is viewed as a geriatric syndrome, a group of symptoms or conditions occurring together in older adults. However, there's no consensus on how best to define or measure frailty.

Medical providers and researchers who work with older adults commonly use two approaches to identifying frailty. One approach is an assessment of physical frailty, an age-related decline in physical functioning affecting several body systems. This includes deficits such as low physical activity, weak grip strength, low energy, slow walking speed and unintended weight loss.

The other approach is what's known as the frailty index, a more general assessment based on the number of health problems an individual has. In addition to the criteria just described, it includes chronic medical conditions, abnormal lab values and difficulties with activities of daily living, such as bathing, dressing and mobility.

Individuals who don't meet the criteria for frailty but display some of the physical deficits are considered pre-frail. They may eventually become frail or, with the right strategies, return to a non-frail state.

While it's uncertain exactly what causes frailty, there's no doubt that several elements or causes are likely involved. There's increasing evidence that impairment in the body's stress response systems, including the immune, endocrine and energy response systems, plays a key role in the development of frailty. Muscle loss (sarcopenia) is also thought to be a major contributor. These changes may be related to a variety of factors, including age-related molecular changes, genetics, chronic environmental exposures and specific diseases.

The bottom line, though, is that the earlier a health care provider can detect indications of frailty, the easier it is to intervene and reverse or slow some of the processes involved. Doctors known as geriatricians are particularly good at recognizing signs of frailty and are familiar with methods to measure it.

RECOVERY FROM INJURY AND AGING

In addition to avoiding frailty, another challenge for older adults is recovering from injury, such as a fall or other accident, or from surgery. As you age, healing and recovery generally take longer and can become more difficult.

An older body faces increased recovery challenges. Your overall health plays a big role in your ability to heal as you age. The following conditions can interfere with your ability to recover. If you're frail, that exacerbates these challenges and can mean longer hospital stays or the need for extended care in another facility.

Loss of bone and muscle mass

As your body ages, it undergoes natural changes that weaken it and make it more susceptible to injury. Muscle wastes away and weakens, bones become less dense, joints become less mobile and connective tissues that hold joints together stiffen and lose flexibility.

Depressed immune system

It remains unclear exactly how getting older interferes with the healing process, but research suggests the immune system plays a key role in its slowdown. It takes longer for your immune cells to respond to your body's call for healing

and for cells to regenerate themselves. Chronic inflammation, which tends to become more common with age, can also reduce your immune response.

Increased blood pressure

Your blood pressure naturally rises with age as your heart rate slows slightly and your arteries become stiffer. This means that your blood circulation may slow somewhat, lowering the amount of oxygen and nutrients distributed throughout your body. Without vigorous circulation, healing is impaired.

Changing sleep patterns

You may have more sleep problems in your senior years. Without proper rest, your body's ability to heal is greatly diminished.

Sedentary lifestyle

Reduced physical activity influences the healing process. A more sedentary lifestyle, common to many older adults, poses several health risks, including obesity, which slows healing because fatty tissue impairs blood flow to other tissues. Fat also suppresses the production of certain substances that protect against inflammation.

Inactivity and reduced mobility during hospitalization can lead to so-called hospital-acquired disability. Generally, the longer the hospital stay and the more time spent in bed, the less your chance of resuming your prior level of functioning on upon discharge.

Nutrition

Older adults may have nutritional deficiencies that can interfere with healing. Some individuals maintain a proper diet but don't eat as much. Older adults are more likely to develop digestive issues that reduce nutrient absorption. Some individuals may eat high-calorie foods that contain few of the

PREHABILITATION: IMPROVING RECOVERY *BEFORE* SURGERY

If you need to have surgery and you're at risk of a prolonged recovery, the good news is that a process called prehabilitation can help. Prehabilitation involves getting you in better shape physically and mentally *prior* to surgery so that you can enjoy a speedier recovery after surgery.

Prehabilitation typically involves exercise and diet but also may include therapies such as muscle relaxation, deep breathing and meditation to reduce surgical-related stress and anxiety.

Prior to knee replacement surgery, for instance, your surgeon may prescribe daily exercises to help strengthen involved muscles, tendons and ligaments. Before cardiac surgery, you may partake in activities to improve your physical health by way of aerobic and strength exercises, breathing exercises, improved nutrition and psychological support.

Studies of individuals who underwent prehabilitation prior to surgery compared with individuals who didn't consistently show improved outcomes and shortened recovery after surgery.

proteins, vitamins and minerals needed to maintain optimal healing.

Vitamin D insufficiency is very common in older adults, especially frail individuals. It can produce a condition called osteomalacia, which causes weak bones, bone pain and muscle weakness. Older adults with vitamin D deficiency are more likely to experience longer recovery times and poorer outcomes after hospitalization.

FRAILTY, RECOVERY AND RESILIENCE

Resilience refers to the capacity to resist or recover from a stress or a challenge. In the context of health, these challenges may be physical, psychological, social or even financial.

Physical resilience includes the capacity to return to normal or to a healthy state after an accident, illness or surgery. Psychological resilience embodies the ability to successfully cope with the losses and adversities that often occur later in life — the psychological aspects of aging. Social and financial resilience involve overcoming factors such as isolation and poverty.

What does resiliency have to do with frailty and recovery? Researchers have found that individuals who are resilient are generally more likely to bounce back after an injury or surgery and less likely to experience frailty.

One way to conceptualize the relationship between frailty and resilience is to view frailty as a vulnerability to major health changes following even minor stresses or events, whereas resilience is the ability to resist and recover from health challenges even in cases of major health problems.

Cultivating a sense of resilience can be a key step in reducing your risk of frailty as you age and improving your recovery after surgery or an injury. And science is showing that the earlier you develop resilient characteristics and the longer you use them, the more resilience you'll have for the inevitable changes and setbacks that come as you get older. Also, the healthier you age, the more optimal your general resilience.

Developing resilience

There are many mental and psychological approaches that can help build resilience. To begin, think about resilient people that you know — people who seem to handle the difficulties and complexities of life in a healthy fashion.

Picture someone you admire, someone you're close to or someone who's overcome challenges. What traits would you use to describe that person? What characteristics does that person have that you would like to cultivate in yourself?

Words often used when describing the characteristics of resilient people include adaptable, calm, grounded, caring, inspirational, peaceful and thoughtful.

How do you develop these characteristics? Tools that can improve your resilience include physical activity and a healthy diet, spending time in healthy environments, practicing positive thinking and developing healthy social relationships. With practice you can become more resilient.

WHAT YOU CAN DO

As mentioned earlier in this chapter, just because you're getting older doesn't mean that you need to become frail. To help prevent frailty, to better equip yourself to recover from injury or illness and to improve your resiliency, following are some strategies to try. You can learn more about many of these approaches in Part 2.

Physical activity

The first and most important strategy is to exercise regularly, making sure to address all major muscle groups. If you generally walk or jog, balance that with some weightlifting, push-ups and sit-ups for the arms and abdominal muscles, respectively.

Exercise is a healthy stress. It can teach the molecules within our cells how to respond to challenges and, importantly, how to return to normal. In a way, exercise is resilience training.

Individuals who exercise regularly are less likely to become frail, and those who are frail can often improve their health with exercise. Exercise counters weakness, slowed mobility, low energy and poor endurance associated with physical frailty; it also prevents other health conditions that can lead to a frailty diagnosis. Regular physical activity and exercise are associated with physical, cognitive and emotional resilience and are, therefore, essential elements of healthy aging.

For older adults who are physically active, at least 150 minutes of exercise a week is recommended. This includes moderately intense aerobic activity and twice-weekly muscle-strengthening exercises. Individuals with chronic conditions who cannot tolerate this recommendation should stay physically active as much as their condition allows.

Dietary strategies to prevent frailty

Aim for three nutritious meals a day that include fruit, vegetables, protein, healthy fats, whole grains and low-fat dairy products. Be sure to include enough muscle-nurturing protein. The daily Recommended Dietary Allowance (RDA) is 0.36 grams per pound of body weight, or 54 grams for a 150-pound person. Many older people don't get this much.

There are indications that as you age, an amount greater than the RDA may be better. This is because as you get older, your body may become less efficient at using protein. Chronic inflammation associated with infection and illness can increase your protein needs. And some medications may pull protein from your muscles if you don't get enough in your diet, decreasing muscle mass and strength.

Good sources of protein include lean meat, fish or poultry; low-fat dairy products; and plant protein such as beans, lentils, nuts, seeds, soy and whole grains. Whey appears to be a particularly good source of protein to build

muscle. Yogurt, cottage cheese and ricotta are rich sources of whey. Ursolic acid, found in apple peels, has also been associated with enhancing muscle mass.

In regard to resiliency, a healthy diet provides important nutrients to help your body better cope with the physical effects of stress, during which times it's common for people to turn to high-calorie comfort foods or snack endlessly on whatever is available.

Benefits of social connections

There's strong evidence that psychological and physical resilience improves with social engagement. We have a natural desire to stay connected with others and to be actively involved in life. Strong social support, social activities, meaningful daily interactions, family life and friendships help build resilience and are good for your overall health.

Relationships are crucial to resiliency; the best single predictor of happiness is the quality of our social relationships. People with emotional support often have lower stress levels, generally enjoy healthier lifestyles and are in better health.

Unfortunately, on life's journey, your social circle can decrease, your friends can move away, your children can leave home, and you can lose your loved ones. That's why taking steps to maintain or enhance your social circle is important. Ways to improve your social connections are discussed in Chapter 13.

Additional strategies

If your goal is to build resilience, consider the following:

- **Your attitude.** While you may not realize it, you talk to yourself all the time. Is what you're telling yourself positive or negative? Throughout the day, be aware of your internal thoughts and keep them positive. Instead of telling yourself, "It will never work," say, "I'm willing to give it a try." Positive thoughts promote self-esteem, and high self-esteem helps build confidence to make healthy changes.
- **Your happiness.** There's a lot of truth behind the idea that happiness is a choice. Even though genetics and life circumstances play a role in your level of happiness, you have control over much of it. It's unrealistic, of course, to snap your fingers and decide to be happy. But if you bring consciousness, gratitude and even frivolity to your day, you'll likely feel more joyful. Find the things that make you happy and spend time doing them.

- **Your mindset.** Your brain is malleable and constantly adjusting. This (thankfully) provides you the ability to learn and adapt with time. Individuals with a growth mindset, as opposed to a fixed one, understand that they can develop their abilities and adapt them to different situations. They realize that setbacks and disappointments are inevitable, helping them to recover more quickly from injury, surgery and unfortunate events.

Awareness of these mental states can improve both mental and physical health.

WHAT DO YOU THINK?

As you reflect on what you just read and contemplate your future health, ask yourself these questions.
- *How do I feel about my current risk of frailty?*
- *What am I doing now that I feel good about?*
- *What are some frailty and recovery risk factors I'd like to improve?*
- *What changes can I make that I'm most likely to stick with?*

Living better
and living longer

How are you doing, and what's your plan?

CHAPTER 12

Now that you've completed the learning phase of this book — understanding how your body changes and the conditions that you're at greater risk of developing with age — it's time to move on to the doing phase. Two important steps to take on your wellness journey are to get a snapshot of your overall health and to strategize about how you can make meaningful changes to your everyday habits that will help you reach your goals.

Healthy aging is a lifelong journey, and there may be times when the task seems overwhelming. However, by having a good plan, you can help reduce potential pitfalls and setbacks.

Most people don't fully appreciate the powerful effect changes to everyday habits can have on their current health, their future health and their quality of life. In some cases, the changes can be lifesaving.

YOUR WELLNESS VISION

Think forward five years into the future, or maybe 10. Imagine you're well and healthy. What would you see? If you took a picture of your life, what's in the picture? Where are you and what are you doing? What's the expression on your face?

The answers to these questions will be different for everyone. One person may envision walking and playing with a grandchild, another may envision relaxing by a pool with a good book in hand and yet another may see friends or family gathered on a typical evening enjoying good food and laughs.

This wellness vision — your road map for healthy aging — doesn't have to be anything big or grandiose. The main thing is that it's a workable plan to help you get or stay healthy so that you can fully enjoy your later years. Think about what you want to see in the future and keep that vision front and center as you assess your current health.

Keep in mind that this chapter is where you can make honest assessments of your overall well-being, your motivation and your ability to make changes. The following refections and questionnaires can help you gauge your physical health. Use this information to help identify areas in which your health is good and those in which you could use some improvement.

SELF-REFLECTION

Before going any further, take time for a bit more self-reflection. As you answer the following questions, think about what you've learned so far about aging and your own personal wellness. You may want to refer back to any notes you may have taken at the end of each of the chapters in Part 1. The information that you gather here is important because it can help you plot a course to health and wellness in your later years.

Why is your health important to you?

_____

_____

_____

How do you envision your overall health a year from now? In five years? In 10 years?

_____

_____

_____

What are you already doing that's good for your health and that you want to continue?

_____

_____

_____

What changes do you feel you need to make to improve your health?

_____
_____
_____

Do you have someone — a friend, family member or coworker — who can support you in your efforts to improve and preserve your health?

_____
_____
_____

On a scale of 1 to 5, with 5 being very confident, how confident are you that you can improve or preserve your health now and in years to come?

_____

PHYSICAL ASSESSMENTS

Now it's time to take stock of your personal health. Following you'll find three questionnaires that you can use to identify areas in which your health is good and areas that need improvement. The questionnaires address your weight and eating habits, your level of fitness and other behaviors that can significantly impact health.

Are your weight and eating habits healthy?

1. *What's your BMI? (Use the chart on page 137.)*
    ☐ Obese (1 point)
    ☐ Underweight or overweight (2 points)
    ☐ Healthy (3 points)

2. *What's your waist measurement? A waist circumference of more than 35 inches for women and more than 40 inches for men indicates increased health risks.*
    ☐ Considerably more than the recommended measurement (1 point)
    ☐ Slightly above the recommended measurement (2 points)
    ☐ At or below the recommended measurement (3 points)

3. *Do you have a health condition that would improve if you lost weight?*
    ☐ Yes (1 point)
    ☐ Possibly (2 points)
    ☐ No (3 points)

4. *Do you eat for emotional reasons, such as when you feel anxious, depressed, stressed, angry or excited?*
    ☐ Always or quite often (1 point)
    ☐ Sometimes (2 points)
    ☐ Never or not often (3 points)

5. *How often do you sit down and eat three regularly scheduled meals?*
   - ☐ Never or not often (1 point)
   - ☐ Sometimes (2 points)
   - ☐ Always or most of the time (3 points)

6. *How long does it generally take you to eat a meal?*
   - ☐ Five minutes or less (1 point)
   - ☐ Between five and 20 minutes (2 points)
   - ☐ 20 minutes or more (3 points)

7. *Do you snack a lot or often have snacks in place of meals?*
   - ☐ Yes or quite often (1 point)
   - ☐ Occasionally (2 points)
   - ☐ No or not often (3 points)

How did you score?

To the right of the answers you chose are point values: 1, 2 and 3 points. Add up the points for your total score.
- If your total score was 18 to 21 points, congratulations! Your weight and eating habits appear to be healthy.
- If your score was 13 to 17 points, you're on track, but you may benefit from losing a few pounds and improving some of your eating habits.
- If your score was 7 to 12 points, prioritize working toward a healthy weight and better eating habits.

Are you fit?

1. *Do you have enough energy to enjoy the leisure activities you like to do?*
   - ☐ Rarely or never (1 point)
   - ☐ Sometimes (2 points)
   - ☐ Always or most of the time (3 points)

2. *Do you have enough stamina and strength to carry out the daily tasks of your life?*
   - ☐ Rarely or never (1 point)
   - ☐ Sometimes (2 points)
   - ☐ Always or most of the time (3 points)

3. *Can you walk a mile without feeling winded or fatigued?*
   - ☐ No (1 point)
   - ☐ Sometimes (2 points)
   - ☐ Yes (3 points)

4. *Can you climb two flights of stairs without feeling winded or fatigued?*
   - ☐ No (1 point)
   - ☐ Sometimes (2 points)
   - ☐ Yes (3 points)

5. *Are you flexible enough to touch your toes?*
   - ☐ No (1 point)
   - ☐ Sometimes (2 points)
   - ☐ Yes (3 points)

6. *Can you carry on a conversation while doing light to moderately*

intense activities, such as brisk walking?

- ☐ No (1 point)
- ☐ Sometimes (2 points)
- ☐ Yes (3 points)

7. *About how many days a week do you spend doing at least 30 minutes of moderately vigorous activity, such as walking briskly or raking leaves?*
- ☐ Zero to two days (1 point)
- ☐ Three to four days (2 points)
- ☐ Five to seven days (3 points)

How did you score?

To the right of the answers you chose are point values: 1, 2 and 3 points. Add up the points for your total score.
- If your total score was 18 to 21 points, congratulations! You're well on your way to overall fitness.
- If your score was 13 to 17 points, you're on the right track, but your activity level could use a little boost.
- If your score was 7 to 12 points, it's time to put getting in shape at the top of your to-do list.

How are your other behaviors?

1. *Do you smoke cigarettes, cigars or pipes or use snuff or chewing tobacco?*

- ☐ Yes (1 point)
- ☐ Very infrequently (2 points)
- ☐ No (3 points)

2. *Do you drink more than a moderate amount of alcohol? (A moderate amount is one drink a day or less for women and two drinks a day or less for men.)*
- ☐ Yes or quite often (1 point)
- ☐ Sometimes (2 points)
- ☐ Never or infrequently (3 points)

3. *Do you see a health care provider for regular checkups?*
- ☐ No (1 point)
- ☐ Sometimes (2 points)
- ☐ Yes (3 points)

4. *Do you wake up multiple times during the night or snore while you're asleep?*
- ☐ Often (1 point)
- ☐ Occasionally (2 points)
- ☐ Never or infrequently (3 points)

5. *How often do you feel sleepy during the day and have trouble functioning because you're tired?*
- ☐ Often (1 point)
- ☐ Occasionally (2 points)
- ☐ Never or infrequently (3 points)

6. *How would you rate your ability to manage daily stress?*

☐ Poor (1 point)
☐ Fair (2 points)
☐ Good (3 points)

7. *How often do you feel lonely, depressed or pessimistic about what's happening around you?*
☐ Often or always (1 point)
☐ Occasionally (2 points)
☐ Never or infrequently (3 points)

8. *How often are you socially active, interacting with other individuals?*
☐ Never or infrequently (1 point)
☐ Occasionally (2 points)
☐ Often or always (3 points)

How did you score?

To the right of the answers you chose are point values: 1, 2 and 3 points. Add up the points from your answers for your total score.

- If your total score was 20 to 24 points, congratulations! You're making wise decisions regarding your health.
- If your score was 14 to 19 points, you're on the right track, but there's room for improvement.
- If your score was 8 to 13 points, your behaviors may be putting your health in jeopardy. Review your responses and select areas where you can try to make improvements.

RESILIENCY ASSESSMENT

As you'll learn in the next chapter, resiliency is an important factor in healthy aging and longevity. To determine your level of resiliency, answer the questions in the chart on the opposite page.

In general, the higher the overall score, the more resilient you are. Note that for questions 1 and 2, having a low score means a higher level of resiliency, while for questions 3 to 10, having a high score means a higher level of resiliency.

You don't have to score a 10 — or a 0 for questions 1 and 2 — to have positive functioning. No one is perfect! For example, if you rate your quality of life as a 7, life is probably pretty good most of the time. But if you rate your quality of life as a 3 or lower, life could probably be better.

CHANGING YOUR BEHAVIORS

Making the decision to adopt a healthier lifestyle isn't easy. The real challenge often comes with putting your words or thoughts into action. According to psychologists who study behavior change, quitting an unhealthy behavior can take anywhere from three to 30

Answer the following questions to determine your baseline resiliency using the following scale: 0 1 2 3 4 5 6 7 8 9 10 (low, never, bad) (high, always, good)	Your score
1. What is your current stress level?	
2. How often do you feel burned out?	
3. In a typical week, how would you rate your energy level away from home?	
4. In a typical week, how would you rate your energy level at home?	
5. After a typical night's sleep, how often do you feel rested?	
6. How would you rate your overall quality of life?	
7. How would you rate your spiritual well-being?	
8. How would you rate your level of support?	
9. How often are you mindful — focused on the present moment?	
10. How would you rate your level of happiness?	
Step 1: Total the scores from questions 1 and 2	___ + ___ = ___
Step 2: Subtract your answer from Step 1 from the number 20.	20 - ___ = ___
Step 3: Total the scores from questions 3 through 10.	___
Step 4: Add your answers from Steps 2 and 3.	___ + ___ = ___
Total score:	___

Source: Mayo Clinic.

tries. And there's no magic bullet for adopting healthier habits. Different techniques work for different people.

But there is good news. By planning your behavior changes carefully and taking small steps, you increase your chances of success. Consider the following strategies.

Be SMART

Set goals for yourself that are **S**pecific, **M**easurable, **A**chievable, **R**elevant and **T**ime-bound. To do this, state exactly what you want to do, how you're going to do it and when you want to achieve it. Start with goals you can achieve within a week or a month.

If you have a big goal, such as stopping smoking, break it down into a series of smaller weekly or daily goals that you can measure. "I want to look better" isn't a good goal because it's not specific and it's hard to measure. "I want to lose five pounds this month" is a better goal because it's specific and measurable.

At the same time, make sure the goals that you set for yourself are achievable and relevant. You may be setting yourself up to fail if you resolve never to eat chocolate again or commit to a two-

hour-a-day fitness regimen, especially if you're relatively new to daily exercise. The test: Can you do this regularly over the long haul? If not, ratchet your goal down a notch.

Schedule and record

You have a better chance of accomplishing your goal — whether it's attending a yoga class or walking three miles — if you put it on your daily calendar. And when you complete a goal, record it somehow — on an app, on a calendar, in a journal, whatever works for you. People who schedule and keep track of their accomplishments are more likely to continue to progress toward their larger goals. One success leads to another!

Share and partner

Going public can give you the peer support — or pressure — you need to succeed. So let friends and family know what you want to accomplish, from learning how to better manage your stress to limiting alcohol. Tell them how they can support you.

You might also ask friends, family or coworkers to join you. You're more likely to go to an aerobics class, eat a healthy lunch, sign up for a smoking cessation class or attend a social event if someone joins you.

Reward yourself

It takes about three months to develop a healthy habit. If you practice it faithfully for that long, you'll be more likely to stay with it for life. When you reach a goal, celebrate. Rewarding yourself with a night out at the movies, a massage from a massage therapist or a new tool for your garage can encourage you to keep up the good work.

Despite what you may think, adopting a healthier lifestyle doesn't have to be a chore. It can, and should, be an enjoyable experience. Many people find that the longer they follow a wellness plan, the easier and more rewarding it becomes. New lifestyle habits gradually replace old ones to create a healthier and happier you!

The power of relationships, connections and purpose

Staying well as you age is about more than your physical health. Human connections and feelings of purpose and contentment are important life factors that contribute to well-being and longevity.

Taking stock of your social and emotional health in your younger years is a good way to start preparing for your later-life journey. What you learn about yourself when evaluating your social and emotional well-being may help you lead a longer and more fulfilling life.

Evaluating your social ties and emotional well-being is an exercise you may want to revisit periodically to ensure that you stay on a healthy course as you get older and life circumstances change.

SOCIAL COMPANIONSHIP AND HEALTH

Relationships are vital to your health and well-being. Throughout life, strong family ties and good friendships contribute to mental and emotional well-being. Studies show that people with good social support — strong relationships with family, friends and partners — not only enjoy better health but live longer.

In a survey by the National Council on Aging, "American Perceptions of Aging in the 21st Century," nearly 90% of respondents thought that having close relationships with family and friends was vital for a meaningful life, ranking higher than many other factors, including health.

The health benefits of friendship

Increasing evidence suggests that physical indicators of your health — your blood cholesterol levels, heart rate, blood pressure and immune system response — are influenced by psychosocial factors, such as your attitude and your relationships. Whereas social isolation can contribute to illness and poor health, having strong connections with the outside world appears to reap many benefits.

Extends life

Several studies link social support with a lower risk of early death. In one study, for example, researchers monitored the health of nearly 7,000 Californians for more than 17 years. They found that those lacking social connections were approximately two and three times more likely to die at a younger age than were their counterparts with more social connections.

Boosts recovery

Researchers who reviewed more than 50 studies examining the association between social support and cardiovascular disease concluded that individuals who don't have the support of family and friends have worse recovery rates after a heart attack. People who enjoy strong social connections may be more motivated to recover and adhere better to treatment regimens. Lack of social support appears to carry the same weight as other cardiovascular risk factors, such as high cholesterol, smoking and high blood pressure.

Bolsters immunity

It's clear that stress can suppress immunity. Love and friendship help to reduce stress. Interestingly, one study found that people with more diverse social networks were less susceptible to the common cold.

Improves mental health

Having people to talk with during difficult times is a psychological buffer against stress, anxiety and depression. Even when you don't have a crisis in your life, social networks increase your sense

In your life journey, you may need to take on the role of care partner. Many of the supportive relationships that we experience with age involve caring for others for an extended period. Families are often the primary source for caregiving. According to the Family Caregiver Alliance, more than 43 million Americans, about 18% of adults, tend to a family member or friend.

Health benefits and risks

The role of care partner can be both deeply rewarding and highly stressful. Caregivers often report that taking on the care of others makes them feel good about themselves. It brings meaning into their lives. In addition to strengthening their emotional bond with their loved one, caregiving offers an opportunity for personal growth.

In one study, researchers from the University of Michigan's Institute for Social Research identified another interesting benefit of caregiving — increased longevity. They found that mortality was "significantly reduced" for individuals who reported providing care to friends, relatives and neighbors and for those who reported providing emotional support to a spouse.

At the same time, caring for a spouse or other loved one or close friend can be very stressful. You may feel as if you've been plunged into a situation that you never asked for and don't feel prepared to execute. Here are some strategies that can help you maintain your own health as you care for others.

Offer empathy. To empathize means to imagine, as best as you can, what it's like to live someone else's life and to seek to understand another person's experience and reality. Showing empathy is good for you and the individual you're caring for. One of the most important things you can do as a care partner is to seek to understand your loved one's experience and reality.

Don't fear negative emotions. The role of caregiver can produce many emotions. Not paying attention to your own feelings can lead to trouble coping with daily life, which can trigger stress eating, increased isolation, depression, substance abuse and more. Experiencing negative emotions doesn't make you a negative person. All feelings are messengers of perception. If you ignore, suppress or deny them, they'll just come out sideways, and that's not always pretty.

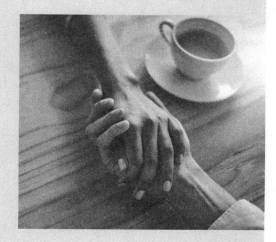

Ask for help. Understand that you don't have to do it all. It's OK to get help from others. Their help can be as valuable to you as to the person you're caring for. Be as specific as you can about the help you need.

Let the doctor take the lead. If your loved one is having trouble accepting certain medical advice, such as taking medications or not driving, let it be the doctor's directive. As a care partner, you need to preserve your relationship with your loved one. It's always better to listen, validate and respond with empathy: "The doctor said you need to stop driving. I'm sorry this is making you upset. This must be hard."

Take care of yourself. During visits with your health care provider, be honest about what you're going through and share any difficult feelings you have. Your provider may be able to offer some helpful advice or to connect you with staff who can. Support groups can be an effective way to manage a host of feelings as you learn from other caregivers. And don't forget the basics — get enough sleep, exercise and eat well.

of belonging and self-worth, promoting positive mental health.

Reduces anxiety

Data suggests that people hospitalized for heart disease who have strong social and religious ties are generally less anxious about upcoming medical events and procedures. Individuals with greater support are less prone to anxiety in general, which, in the case of cardiovascular disease, is associated with increased risk of mortality and sudden cardiac death.

Protects against mental decline

One mind can sharpen another. A study of older adults living in Spain found that having multiple social ties ranging from intimate to extended, maintaining frequent contact with these individuals and involving the individuals in their lives helped to preserve mental ability.

Another study examining the link between social networks and mental sharpness found that participants who frequently interacted with larger networks, such as civic and church groups, were more likely to stay mentally sharp over time.

Finding the link

It's clear that social connections impact individual health. The question becomes how or why. There's still much to learn, but researchers suspect that personal relationships:
- Reduce stress.
- Motivate individuals to engage in healthy behaviors, such as walking regularly or quitting smoking.
- Result in direct expressions of affection, esteem and respect (socioemotional support), which may increase biological resistance to disease.
- Allow for timely medical care and access to personal care if needed.
- Lead to practical help when needed — for example, assistance with daily chores and transportation.

HOW TO BUILD A SUPPORT NETWORK

Casual friendships may come and go, but most people have a group of friends and family they can turn to when they need support. The members of this inner circle may change over time, but the number usually remains fairly stable during the course of a lifetime.

To build and maintain a strong network of family and friends, invest in some key relationship strategies:

- **Make relationships a priority.** A healthy, fulfilling long-term relationship is one of the best sources of support. Don't take your partner or spouse for granted. Take time to be there for each other, and also make time to regularly do something with your friends.
- **Recognize the importance of give-and-take.** Sometimes you're the one giving support, and other times you're on the receiving end. Letting family and friends know you love and appreciate them will help ensure that their support remains strong when times are rough for you.
- **Respect boundaries.** Although you want to be there for friends and family, you don't want to overwhelm them. Respect their ways of communicating. Find out how often they like to get together.
- **Don't compete.** This can turn potential rivals into potential friends.
- **Avoid relentless complaining.** Nonstop complaining is tiresome and can be draining on others.
- **Embrace laughter.** Try to find the humor in things.
- **Listen up.** Make a point to remember what's going on in others' lives. Relate any interests or experiences you have in common.
- **Resolve to improve yourself.** Cultivating your own honesty, generosity and

humility will enhance your self-esteem and make you a more compassionate and appealing friend.
- **Beware of individuals or groups that are unhealthy, oppressive or rigid.** They can be just as damaging as having no connections at all. For instance, if people in your social support system are continually stressed or ill, you may end up suffering along with them. If your friends place heavy demands on your time, or if you're unable to meet their needs, you may find yourself become increasingly anxious or depressed. You may pay a psychological price if you feel obligated to conform to your friends' beliefs or ideas.

RESILIENCY, OPTIMISM AND HEALTH

Life, as you know, isn't perfect. Events often don't go as planned or hoped. Days can be hectic, unpredictable or stressful. On your aging journey, you're bound to encounter negative experiences, difficult losses and stressful situations. Depending on how you cope with these events, they can have a negative or positive effect on your health, relationships and quality of life.

Studies have found that people who are more resilient to life's challenges — who are able to bounce back quickly and grow from their experiences — tend to be healthier and happier. Are you a resilient person? If not, can you learn to be more resilient? The answer is yes.

Research suggests that strategies used to reduce stress — physical activity, a healthy diet, relaxation techniques — also bolster resiliency. (For more on resiliency see pages 182-185.) Your daily environment also is important. For example, if you spend all day in a sterile environment running laboratory tests, offset that with activities and events that allow you to be around other individuals and socialize. In contrast, if you're a teacher and are talking to people all day long, at the end of your day a nice walk alone outdoors might be exactly what you need.

Finally, resiliency is closely tied to your view on life. If you approach life's events with a positive, optimistic attitude, you're more likely to weather life's ups and downs and make positive lifestyle changes over time. Being optimistic doesn't mean you're always happy or you expect good things will always happen to you. Yes, optimistic people are often happy and positive, but more importantly, when bad things happen, their mindset provides the skills and support to overcome them.

Optimists live longer

Increasing evidence suggests that being an optimist or a pessimist affects your health. A Dutch study found that older adults with an optimistic disposition — people who generally expected good things rather than bad things to happen — lived longer than those who tended to expect doom and gloom.

After accounting for factors such as age, sex, smoking, alcohol consumption, physical activity, and socioeconomic and marital status, those in the study who scored high on the optimism scale had a 29% lower risk of early death than did individuals who scored lower on the scale.

In this study, a positive outlook appeared to be particularly protective against death from cardiovascular problems. Highly optimistic participants were 77% less likely to die of a heart attack, stroke or other cardiovascular event than were highly pessimistic participants. These results held true regardless of whether the participants had a history of cardiovascular disease or high blood pressure.

A Mayo Clinic study found similar results. Researchers examined the relationship between how adults explained the causes of life's events and their mortality rate over a 30-year period. They found that individuals who were more pessimistic died younger than did those who were more optimistic.

Optimists tended to believe factors associated with bad events were temporary, not their fault and limited to the present circumstances. Pessimists, on the other hand, were more likely to blame things on themselves, feel that their current situation was going to last forever and feel that a bad event would undermine everything.

Optimists live better

Using the same group of people, Mayo researchers examined the association between outlook on life events and self-reported health status 30 years later. Optimists generally reported fewer health limitations and problems with work or other daily routines, less pain, more energy and greater ease with social activities. They were also more peaceful, happier and calmer most of the time.

Other studies suggest that optimists are less likely to experience coronary artery disease, and if they do undergo heart surgery, their recovery and health afterward are better.

Individuals who are pessimists, on the other hand, have been found to be more prone to depression, have weaker immune systems and use more medical and mental health care services.

Finding the link

Scientists aren't sure exactly how optimism benefits health or how pessimism can translate into poorer health and earlier death. In the Dutch study, optimists were associated with higher levels of physical activity, moderate alcohol use, less smoking, a higher educational level and living with a spouse. But even after adjusting for these factors, optimism still had an independent effect on the death rate.

Part of the explanation may be that optimists, by their very nature, tend to report better health. However, the Dutch study found that optimists lived longer than pessimists, even if they had chronic illnesses or physical disabilities.

It's possible that the habits of optimists, such as taking medications as prescribed or following a treatment regimen, are more likely to promote health and recovery. Biological factors related to immune system health, hormones and genetics may also be involved.

TRANSITIONS AND HEALTH

Change is a part of life and a natural circumstance of aging. Whether change is voluntary or involuntary — or a little bit of both — most of us can handle it in small doses, such as switching an exercise class from Monday to Thursday. Transitions, on the other hand, can profoundly alter your way of life, so much that you may need to develop new dimensions of your identity to cope.

Marriage is a classic example. You go from being single and responsible for only your welfare to being a partner in a relationship in which you generally share goals, interests, responsibilities and usually living quarters. Establishing a successful and loving relationship with another person requires compromise, and that almost always means changing your individual habits. Even if many of these changes are small, together they may seem significant.

Other examples of life transitions include becoming a parent, changing careers, relocating to a different community, retiring from the workforce, developing a chronic illness, caring for a loved one, losing a family member or friend and separating or getting a divorce from a partner. In all of these, the changes involved become part of a transformative process, a move from one phase of your life to another.

It's important to note that there is a difference between anticipated endings — the ones that are planned and often less traumatic — and unanticipated endings. Unanticipated endings can be much more difficult to accept and manage, and you may need different transitional skills to cope with them.

William Bridges, who explores the concept of transition in his books, describes the transitional process as beginning with an ending, followed by a middle or "neutral zone," and finally reaching a new beginning after a period of adjustment. So, although it may seem self-contradictory, transition typically starts with an end — some form of loss.

Take retirement, for example. It may be something that you've happily anticipated, but on that first free day, you may not be quite sure what to do or who you are without your work identity. If your partner or spouse is the one who retires and is now around a lot more, this may disrupt your usual routine and take some getting used to.

Major life transitions entail even bigger losses and adjustments. The death of a partner or spouse can be overwhelming because it represents the loss of the familiar and of future plans and dreams.

When you experience the end of a chapter in your life, it's important to acknowledge the losses that accompany it, no matter how great or small. The only way to reach the next phase is through the passage of time, and during the middle period of transition, you may feel anxious, uneasy and vulnerable.

Transition also offers opportunity. Take time to pause and rediscover what's meaningful to you. Step back and reflect on your priorities and interests. As you gain confidence in your new beginning, don't be afraid to take pleasure in it. You won't be discrediting what you may have lost, such as a long and fulfilling career. Rather, you'll be affirming the power of your past experiences to help you become a healthy, strong and vibrant person.

PURPOSE AND HEALTH

The second half of your life can be interesting, fulfilling and exciting, or it can be frustrating, boring and depressing. The difference is in the choices you make. Your later years offer an abundance of opportunities to learn, explore and share.

However, your goal shouldn't be to just keep busy. You want to take part in activities that are meaningful to you — that engage your mind, body and soul and motivate you to get up every morning — in other words, activities that are purposeful.

Purpose is important. Having a sense of purpose helps instill optimism and keeps you from looking back on your life and saying, "What happened?" As Mark Twain observed, you'll have regrets and remorse for the things you didn't do rather than for what you did.

A sense of purpose can mean different things to different people. For many people, it's the feeling that they matter — others depend on them, are interested in them and are concerned about what happens to them. For some, it's spending time doing things that have meaning and that help them feel better about themselves.

To find satisfaction and fulfillment in your later years, you need to figure out what's important to you. The more you take part in activities that you find meaningful, the more you'll enjoy this stage of your life.

Your health will benefit, too. That's because study after study shows that purposeful activities, along with close relationships, improve quality of life.

Data from the Health and Retirement Study show that people over age 50 who engage in leisure activities — who have something to do that they look forward to — are less likely to feel sad and unhappy. Without a sense of mission — a passion for something or someone — you may become vulnerable to depression and other health concerns.

A challenging event for many people is making the transition to retirement. A meta-analysis of five decades of research showed that purposeful social connections and physical health were strongly associated with how well people adjusted to retirement. Surprisingly, those two factors had an even greater impact than finances, retirement planning or how people exited their work.

Finding your purpose

If you're concerned that life isn't purposeful enough, you may wonder how to find greater purpose. There isn't any magic formula for this. Doing things that you enjoy is paramount. To help steer you in the right direction for the next phase of your life you might make a "wish list."

Take time to dream

Ask yourself a few questions: "Who do I want to be for the rest of my life?" "What are my values?" "How can I use my skills?" "What's really important to me?" Your later years can be a time to live unfulfilled dreams or develop underused talents.

Write down activities you see yourself doing

Try to include more than just solitary pursuits, such as reading, watching TV or walking. A list heavy on material things, such as buying a new "toy" or redecorating your house, may not be satisfying for long, either.

Be specific

Many people have a few general ideas about what they'd like to do in their later years, such as traveling, taking classes or spending more time golfing or playing pickleball. If you focus on a specific idea, such as creating a family website or starting a landscaping business, there might be steps you can take now toward that goal to help support your success when you're ready to retire.

Share your thoughts

Talk to your partner or spouse about your ideas. Do you both have the same goals for socializing, travel, finances and so on in retirement? Look for overlapping interests. Talk about areas that may not fit well together and discuss how you'll resolve them.

Consider your finances

Retirement is a major life event, and your income and budget are likely to change. Plan ahead for this so that in your retirement you can achieve your goals and aren't hampered by financial concerns.

Test your ideas

It's a good idea to do a reality check of your ideas. Some people unexpectedly find themselves bored with the activities they planned. Or they find that it's more difficult than they anticipated to start a new business or find an interesting part-time job.

If you can, make time in midlife to get some hands-on experience with the activities you imagine yourself doing in retirement. You may think you'll enjoy consulting or volunteering, but that's just a guess until you actually try it. In addition, unless you have some experience, you may not be able to get the job or volunteer position you want.

If you're thinking of turning a hobby, such as gardening, into a business, you'll need small-business skills. You might want to take classes that will prepare you to run a small business as well as talk to other people who've done something similar to see if you're up to the effort involved.

If you hope to keep working in some capacity — in your field or in a new career — take an inventory of your interests, talents and achievements, and brainstorm ways to build on them. It's important to create and maintain a network of friends and colleagues who may be able to help you.

Talk to people you admire

Finding retirement role models — people who have retired successfully and are energized and satisfied in life — can be helpful as you plan for your later years. Ultimately, each of us must forge our own path, but you can learn from people who've gone before you. Make time to visit with them.

Pursue new hobbies and interests

Your 40s and 50s are a good time to consider finding a hobby that intrigues you, if you don't already have one. What intellectual or physical pursuits do you find fascinating, fun or pleasurable? The list might include cooking, gardening, reading, woodworking, playing bridge or tinkering in the garage, to name a few.

Be realistic about your expectations. If you're trying something new or learning something complex, start simple and build from there. If you take on too much too soon, you may become frustrated and disillusioned and want to quit.

Take a class

You're never too old to learn. Learning provides mental stimulation that helps keep your brain healthy. Studies on aging show that individuals with higher levels of education do better later in life

---

WORKAMPING: RVING FOR FUN AND PROFIT

If you've always dreamed of hitting the road in a recreational vehicle (RV) when you retire but want to continue earning an income, workamping may be for you.

Workampers are adults who live in RVs and supplement their savings or retirement funds by taking seasonal jobs. There are no official statistics on this aspect of the workforce, but numbers seem to be growing with the increase in gig-type employment. According to Workamper News, which has been published since 1987, workampers work not only in campgrounds but also in several other capacities, including as utility inspectors, flea market assistants and craft vendors.

A 2022 survey of subscribers to the publication showed that 46% of active workampers were ages 61 to 70, and 78% were full-time RVers. The typical length of a job taken by the respondents was four to five months, and just over half received hourly pay plus a rent-free RV site.

than people who don't fully develop their intellectual capacities.

A class can help you refresh old skills or develop new ones, especially because technology changes so quickly. It gives you a chance to study for the sheer joy of learning. If you're like most adults, you went to school earlier in life to get work-related skills. For some people, that education may have been interrupted because of family or work responsibilities.

Consider a part-time job

Many people who enjoy the challenges and social interactions of the workplace want to keep working at least part time after retiring. Paid employment may be a good option if you need the income or want to stretch your retirement funds. The right job can also boost your self-esteem and add to your quality of life. In addition to providing regular contact with people, work can give you a feeling of being needed and of contributing — a sense of purpose.

You don't necessarily have to keep doing the same type of work. Maybe you want to try something new, perhaps something that aligns with your hobbies or outside interests.

Volunteer

Many people find community service and volunteering very fulfilling. A lot of nonprofit organizations wouldn't survive if it weren't for dedicated volunteers.

By volunteering your time and talents, you're also helping yourself. For decades, research has shown a link between quality of life and involvement with others. Regular volunteering can improve your physical and psychological well-being and may even help you live longer. Most individuals who volunteer say they feel like they're making a positive difference, feel needed and valued and feel better about themselves and the world around them.

Other benefits of volunteering include staying busy and productive and making new friends. Volunteering can also increase your sense of belonging within a community.

Numerous volunteer options are likely available in your community. Places that often need volunteers include hospitals, schools, libraries, food banks, scout troops, religious organizations, parks, environmental programs, historic sites and organizations for children and youth. Check out the organizations of interest to you.

Express your creativity

Your later years are an excellent time to discover, revisit or hone artistic impulses. Many artists experience a burst of sustained creativity after age 65. Being more creative — drawing, painting, writing, sculpting, sewing, dancing, singing, taking photos, acting, making a video, playing an instrument or composing music — enhances your enjoyment of life and gives it meaning.

SPIRITUALITY AND HEALTH

In addition to a strong support network and an optimistic attitude, a number of scientific studies suggest that the quality of your life and your ability to cope with stress and adversity in your later years is influenced by your spiritual well-being. Like optimism and social support, a strong sense of spirituality is important to both your mental and physical health.

MAINTAINING YOUR IDENTITY

Individuals who are married or have partners often face new challenges in their later years. You may find yourself spending a lot more time with your partner or spouse than you used to. That can be difficult if you don't find a balance between the interests you both share and your individual hobbies and pursuits.

Having hobbies and social activities separate from those of your partner or spouse gives you established ties that you can rely on in the unfortunate event something should happen to your significant other. Plus, your partner or spouse may not be interested in the same things you are. For example, perhaps you've been looking forward to doing a lot of traveling after retirement — but your significant other hates to fly. One solution is for you to travel with friends or a group.

The more you can prepare ahead of time for when you and your spouse or partner spend time together in retirement, the less anxiety you're likely to experience when big life transitions come knocking at your door.

Defining spirituality

People often use the words *spirituality* and *religion* interchangeably. There's considerable overlap between the two concepts, but the terms aren't necessarily synonymous.

Religion typically refers to a formal system of beliefs, attitudes or practices held by a group of believers, whereas *spirituality* is more individualistic and self-determined.

There may be as many definitions of *spirituality* as there are people in the world. One common definition is "a personal search for meaning and purpose in life."

Many people consider themselves to be spiritual and religious. Spirituality and religion both push you to turn inward and reflect on your own life and its purpose. Your spiritual beliefs can help you prioritize your life and develop interests that have the potential to be most fulfilling.

Spiritual and religious beliefs may also help you to connect to something larger than yourself. This may include the divine, people around you, humanity in general, art or music, the natural world or all of the above.

What research shows

The relationship between religion, spirituality and mental and physical health is garnering increasing medical attention. More studies are suggesting that when you believe in something larger than yourself, you strengthen your ability to cope with whatever life hands you.

People who attend religious services tend to enjoy better health, live longer and recover from illness faster and with fewer complications than do those who don't attend such services. They also tend to cope better with illness and experience less depression.

Finding the link

Researchers aren't quite sure of the mechanisms by which religion and spirituality promote mental and physical health. Here are some factors thought to play a role.

Social support

Whether you attend church, synagogue or mosque, these religious settings usually have a built-in social support structure that's readily available to members. Plus, most religious congregations offer assistance — emotional, spiritual and practical — such as meals and housing. Faith communities also offer opportunities for friendship.

Having religious social ties may be especially helpful for easing transitions such as children leaving home, retirement or the death of a partner or spouse. In addition, as people age, they may depend on fellow members to help them with household tasks, shopping or transportation.

Coping resources

Your religious beliefs may help you make sense of the world around you, especially during times of crisis or when tragedies arise. Turning to God or another higher power for comfort and strength may provide relief from stressors in life that can have a negative impact on your health. In addition, the feeling of hope, prominent in many faiths, may boost your immune system.

Belief in something larger than yourself may help you accept and cope with events beyond your control. By learning to accept things that can't be changed, you're able to devote more energy to events in your life that you can control.

Social regulation

Research suggests that people who belong to religious communities are less likely to smoke or abuse alcohol or drugs, more inclined to view physical activity as a priority and less likely to carry or use weapons, get into fights or engage in risky sexual behavior than are individuals who do not.

Forgiveness

The practice of forgiveness is prominent in religion. There's evidence that forgiving others promotes mental and physical well-being, possibly by:
- Relieving the burden of pent-up anger and resentment.
- Reestablishing social ties that may have been a major source of support.
- Promoting positive emotions, which can reduce anxiety and blood pressure.

Prayer

One survey on prayer found that around 90% of Americans pray, and a large number do so at least once a day. It's believed that engaging in rituals such as prayer or meditation promotes relaxation, resulting in lower blood pressure and reduced heart, breathing and metabolic rates. This may have a protective effect, particularly against high blood pressure.

DEVELOPING YOUR SPIRITUALITY

Going through life transitions can affect your awareness of spiritual matters and bring your spiritual needs into focus. At a basic level, spirituality is linked to self-discovery and the development of your inner self. It's an evolving process, based on your upbringing, personality and experiences.

Attending religious services, joining a charitable organization and volunteering in your community are a few ways to express and expand your spiritual side. Many people find these activities bring an added sense of purpose to their lives as they put their time and talents to positive use.

Prayer and meditation are common expressions of spirituality. Sometimes, just shutting off the computer or television and sitting quietly can help you get in touch with inner thoughts and feelings. Writing down your thoughts can help you sort them out and allows you to reexamine them later. Still other people find inner spirituality — what they often

term inner peace — through music, dance, art or exploration of nature.

To help you gain a better understanding of yourself and become more acquainted with your spiritual side, ask yourself the following questions:

- What gives my life meaning and purpose?
- What gives me hope?
- How do I get through tough times? In what circumstances do I generally find comfort?
- What are the three most memorable experiences in my life so far?
- How have I survived previous losses and transitions in my life?
- What helps me get through the daily grind?
- When (a particular time or instance) did I feel life was particularly meaningful? What caused me to feel that way?
- Was there a time when I was filled with a sense of awe?

A FEW FINAL THOUGHTS

Simply thinking happy thoughts or having a large circle of friends won't prevent or cure a serious illness. But research suggests that people who tend to do well when faced with a health condition often share a number of characteristics. These characteristics include:

- A partner or advocate who connects with them and can speak on their behalf.
- A sense of community — whether it's faith-based, work-based or simply the camaraderie of friends — for support and encouragement.
- An acknowledgment that life isn't always fair and that the good guys don't always win balanced with an equal understanding that we each have gifts to share.
- Some element of spirituality — belief in a power or an energy beyond oneself that can be a source of comfort and strength.

While not a quick recipe for a long and healthy life, these key ingredients may help you make the best of the life you're living.

Improving your physical health with exercise

Wouldn't it be great if we could make major lifestyle changes with just a flip of a switch, perhaps coupled with a little bit of willpower? But we might as well be honest — that expectation isn't logical or reasonable.

Think of all the people who each year join fitness centers or buy shiny new exercise equipment with the best of intentions. But after one or two workouts, they pull a muscle, injure a joint or lose their enthusiasm, and they can't bring themselves to return to the gym or step back on that fitness machine.

The same thing happens when we try to change our eating patterns. At any one time, nearly half of all adults in the U.S. are attempting to lose weight. By making dramatic changes to what and how much they eat, many of them succeed. The problem is that those big, sudden changes typically don't stick. Over time, most people gain the weight back and then some. So what's the answer? Small changes over time.

Experience suggests that the fastest way to create a lasting habit is to go slow. How can going slow be fast? Think of the moral from the fable about the tortoise and the hare: Slow and steady wins the race. We're more likely to succeed when we make small changes over a long period of time.

Recommendations on how to improve health and longevity are generally nothing that you haven't heard before: Exercise, eat healthy, don't smoke, get enough sleep, limit stress and so forth. Like a lot of people, you may know what you need to do; the problem is that you have trouble getting from point A to point B — from knowing to doing.

Successful change generally begins with powerful motivation, which is different from willpower. Ask yourself, "Why should I get more exercise?" or "Why do I need to stop stressing so much?" And really think about it. What's your driving force?

In general, positive motivations are more effective than negative ones. Guilt, shame or fear likely won't inspire you for the long haul. Instead of being inspired by fear of a heart attack, for example, your motivator might be to see a grandchild graduate or to have enough energy and mobility to travel the world.

To reach your goals, focus on your habits. Our habits control at least half of what we do every day. A change in habit is the best way to improve your lifestyle and your health. The key is to take it slow: one change in habits at a time.

A KEY STEP

Good old-fashioned sweat-inducing exercise is probably the *single most important thing* that you can do to live well. Read that sentence again! Even in moderate amounts, exercise can help you better enjoy life and prevent diseases that people mistakenly believe automatically come with age.

Almost anyone can exercise. Few people are too old, too young, too sick, too poor or too busy to be physically active. Exercise is an equal-opportunity activity. With exercise, people with chronic conditions can improve their stamina, mental outlook and ability to perform daily tasks. Older adults can use strength training to combat the problems of osteoporosis and age-related loss of muscle mass (sarcopenia).

People of any age who say they're too tired to exercise often find they have increased energy after just a few sessions of physical activity. Truth be told, very few people have a valid excuse for not engaging in some form of exercise.

By introducing a moderate amount of physical activity into your daily life, you can significantly improve your overall health, well-being and quality of life. The activity you choose to do is up to you, but try to include both aerobic activity and resistance training. And keep in mind, the more you exercise, the more you may benefit. If you're already getting 30 minutes of physical activity a day, adding one more mile to your daily walk or taking the stairs instead of the elevator can make your heart, muscles and lungs even healthier.

Whether you're 25 or 85, regular repetitive physical activity can provide the benefits you need to help you look and feel better and enjoy great health.

Activity and health

Many of your basic bodily functions start to decline at a rate of about 1% to 2% a year after age 30. This is an undeniable fact of the aging process. But with exercise, you can slow this decline to a rate of about half a percent a year.

Consider this example: People who don't get any physical activity lose about 70% of their functional ability by the time they reach age 90. On the flip side, individuals who exercise regularly lose only 30% of their functional ability by that age.

When you move about, your muscles squeeze or contract to help you walk, run, jump or swing your arms. When muscles contract, they stimulate an anti-inflammatory response set in motion by your immune system. Inflammation, as you'll recall from Chapter 1, can exist at a low-level, chronic state in the body and contribute to different diseases.

Regular physical activity, including exercise, helps keep inflammation in check. It halts or slows circulation of pro-inflammatory compounds such as interleukins, cytokines and others in the bloodstream that can damage the lining of your arteries, resulting in stiff artery walls, plaque formation and increased blood pressure.

Physical activity, especially resistance training, keeps your body sensitive to the effects of insulin, the hormone that regulates blood sugar levels. You want your cells to be receptive to insulin so that you don't have high levels of the hormone traveling through your bloodstream. Too much insulin can lead to inflammation and damage the lining of your arteries. This is what happens with type 2 diabetes.

Plus, exercise helps prevent excess body fat. When too much fat accumulates, it ends up getting stored in inappropriate places, such as your liver and abdomen. Excess body fat wreaks havoc on your body, creating a toxic effect on cells that eventually causes cell death and in some circumstances can lead to organ failure.

What's in it for you?

Beyond the physiological changes associated with increased activity, these are some of the ways that exercise helps you feel healthier and look younger.

Keeps your body firm

Regular exercise — particularly resistance training — slows the loss of muscle mass and strengthens your muscles as you age. Muscles naturally lose their tone and texture (elasticity) with time. As your muscles become stiff and sag from the constant pull of gravity, your body begins to show signs of aging. As muscle mass declines, your percentage of body fat increases. This is a primary driver of frailty and falls.

By engaging in a regular resistance training program, you can maintain your

---

PHYSICAL ACTIVITY VS. EXERCISE

The terms *physical activity* and *exercise* are used throughout this book. And although they're closely related — and often overlap — there is a difference. *Physical activity* refers to any body movement that burns calories, such as mowing the lawn, doing laundry or walking the dog. Exercise refers to a more structured form of physical activity. It involves a series of repetitive movements designed to strengthen or develop some part of your body and improve your cardiovascular fitness. *Exercise* includes walking, swimming, bicycling and many other activities.

Exercise is a form of physical activity, but not all physical activity fits the definition of *exercise*. The good news is that you can gain health benefits through regular physical activity, even if it's not in the form of structured exercise.

muscle mass and tone and counteract the effects of gravity. As a result, you'll look younger longer. You'll also better maintain your strength and day-to-day functioning.

Gives you energy

Many people complain that they don't have the energy to do the things they once did. They assume that their lack of energy is a result of their age, when it's largely the result of inactivity.

Endurance exercises, such as walking, swimming, jogging, biking and rowing, improve stamina and energy. After just a few weeks in a walking program, for instance, most people find they have more energy to do things such as gardening, traveling and spending time

A CURE FOR THE COMMON COLD?

Regular activity may boost your immune system. Researchers have found a link between exercise and improved immune function. During moderate exercise, immune cells circulate more quickly through your body and are better at destroying viruses and bacteria.

Researchers at the University of South Carolina in Columbia investigated the relationship between different levels of physical activity and the risk of getting a cold (upper respiratory tract infection). The study included 547 healthy adults between the ages of 20 and 70. Those who took part in moderate to high levels of physical activity experienced 20% to 30% fewer colds than did those whose levels of daily activities were low.

Moderation is key. Some studies have found that intense physical training may lead to a suppressed immune system and increased susceptibility to illness. Running a marathon, for example, may deplete your immune system defenses and leave you vulnerable to colds and other illnesses during the week after the race.

with friends or grandchildren. Taking part in resistance training to offset the loss of muscle mass that comes with age can have a similar effect.

Encourages mental well-being

Exercise can provide both a direct and an indirect boost to your mental state. There's considerable evidence that regular physical activity can help reduce stress, manage mild to moderate depression and anxiety, improve sleep, boost your mood and enhance your self-image and overall sense of well-being.

Reduces stress

According to the Society of Behavioral Medicine, people who participate in high levels of physical activity may actually reduce the amount of stress they experience — using exercise as a stress buffer. Here's how:

- **Exercise is relaxing and soothing.** Even as you exert your body during physical activity, your mind maintains a sense of calm and control. You may feel in comand of your body and your life, and experience a heightened sense of well-being. It's no wonder many people who exercise regularly have normal blood pressure even under stress.

- **Exercise provides a positive coping strategy.** Physical activity offers a sort of time-out from the problems and stressors of everyday life. While exercising, you tend to concentrate on the task at hand — pushing it one more mile, for example — and not the tensions of your day. People who exercise are generally better able to cope with stress and, according to research, are less likely to be depressed and anxious.

Combats depression

People who are inactive are generally twice as likely to experience symptoms of depression as people who are physically active. Why is that? Exercise fights depression by activating brain neurotransmitters — chemicals used by your nerve cells to communicate with one another. When you experience depression, the level of the neurotransmitters serotonin or norepinephrine may be out of balance. Exercise may lessen the risk of depression by helping to synchronize these brain chemicals.

Exercise also stimulates the production of endorphins — other neurotransmitters that produce feelings of well-being. This phenomenon is commonly referred to as runner's high, but you don't have to run to get it. Many people will feel this uplifting rush just 12 minutes into a workout. One study found that depressed people experienced significantly less depression after exercising for 20 minutes to an hour three times a week for five weeks.

Another study suggested that exercise may stimulate growth of new brain cells that enhance memory and learning — two functions hampered by depression. It has even been suggested that regular physical activity may prevent or reduce the risk of developing depression and some forms of dementia, although further research is needed.

Reduces anxiety

People who experience anxiety often feel tense, nervous and apprehensive of something they can't define. Anxiety is an ongoing tension with negative health effects.

INACTIVITY CAN BE DEADLY

Our ancestors didn't have formal exercise programs. Time spent laboring in fields or factories, or cooking, cleaning and gardening kept them active. Compared to just five decades ago, people today move less. At work, we sit at our desks for hours. At home we're less active, where it's all too tempting to park ourselves in front of the TV or shop online instead of going to a store.

All of that inactivity adds up. On average, we spend half our days sitting, and it's taking a toll. Prolonged periods of sitting are associated with an increased risk of health problems such as diabetes, heart disease and some cancers — not to mention weight gain and obesity.

Increased physical fitness has been shown to counter the negative effects of many risk factors associated with inactivity. In one study, for instance, moderately fit smokers with high cholesterol lived longer than did healthy but inactive nonsmokers.

Physical activities such as walking have been shown to reduce chronic anxiety for the same reasons that exercise helps manage mild or moderate depression. Exercise also serves as a diversion, giving an anxious mind a break — and a chance to refocus. One study found that a single session of exercise — in this case, walking — was just as effective as a prescribed tranquilizer in reducing tension. In addition, the benefit of the exercise lasted longer.

Improves mood and self-esteem

When you exercise, you're being proactive — you're taking control of your life and health. You'll improve your strength, endurance and appearance. You may even lose weight. As a result, you'll feel better about yourself. This new confidence will carry over into your everyday life — improving your outlook.

Enhances sleep

A good night's sleep helps maintain both your physical and mental health. Exercise can help you get much-needed rest. Studies show that moderate exercise, when done at least three hours before bedtime, can help you relax and sleep better at night.

Prevents disease

One of the greatest myths about health is that illness is an inevitable part of aging. This isn't true. Although illness and disease do occur more often as people get older, this is as much a result of inactivity and other lifestyle factors as it is age. Regular exercise helps you reduce, prevent or slow many diseases and disorders.

How much exercise is enough?

A friend says her doctor told her 30 minutes of exercise three days a week is effective. A magazine you picked up last week claims you need to be physically active at least five days a week. And a story on the news last night said everyone should get 90 minutes of physical activity every day.

The answer to the question, "How much is enough?" will change over the course of your life. The amount of exercise you need is based on some widely accepted guidelines and your specific goals.

Most healthy adults need at least 150 minutes of moderate aerobic activity or 75 minutes of vigorous aerobic activity a week, or a combination of moderate and vigorous activity. You can spread out this exercise during the course of a week. That translates to about 30 minutes a day most days of the week.

However, additional benefits generally occur with more physical activity — beyond 150 minutes a week. This is especially true for adults trying to lose weight or get control of certain chronic health conditions, such as diabetes or high blood pressure.

It's also important to include resistance training in your exercise routine. It's recommended you perform resistance training exercises for all major muscle groups at least twice a week. Activities that promote flexibility and balance, such as yoga and tai chi, are also beneficial, especially as you get older.

AEROBIC EXERCISE

Aerobic exercise includes activities during which oxygen plays an important role in the release of energy in your muscles. Aerobic exercise involves some of the most common exercises you'll do. Examples include walking, dancing, biking and swimming, all at a low to moderately intense pace.

No matter what your age, aerobic exercise will help you in your daily activities. It will help your heart, blood vessels, lungs and muscles complete routine tasks and rise to unexpected challenges. It will improve your stamina and endurance so that you can do the things you want to, whether it's training for a marathon or playing hide-and-seek with your grandchildren.

Almost any activity you do — whether it's taking a walk, doing the dishes or walking up stairs — requires oxygen. When your aerobic capacity is high, your heart, lungs and blood vessels efficiently transport and deliver large amounts of oxygen throughout your body. As a result, you don't fatigue as quickly. If you don't get enough aerobic exercise, your aerobic capacity is reduced, and you fatigue more easily.

Aerobic exercise also burns calories to help you lose weight or maintain a healthy weight, and it can increase your life span and improve the overall function of your body.

The key to enjoying and maintaining aerobic activity is to select activities that you enjoy and can do regularly. You don't need to limit yourself to a single activity — a variety is often better. No matter what you do, the idea is to start slowly and then work up to a more intense pace as you feel ready.

GETTING STARTED ON A WALKING PROGRAM

Walking is an excellent relatively low-impact exercise. It's simple, inexpensive and versatile and requires no equipment other than a good pair of shoes.

If you're a seasoned walker, keep doing what you're doing. If you've been inactive and become fatigued easily, it's best to start slow and easy. At first, walk only as far or as fast as you find comfortable. For example, you might try short daily sessions of 10 minutes and slowly build up to 15 minutes twice a week. Then gradually increase the pace of your workout over a period of 4 to 6 weeks.

For the first few weeks, walk on paths over flat, level ground. As you progress, try adding routes that include hills to increase the intensity of your workout.

Use the chart below as a guide to increasing the intensity of your walking program.

	Distance	Time
Week 1	1-2 miles	15-30 min./mile
Week 2	1-2 miles	15-30 min./mile
Week 3	2-2½ miles	13-25 min./mile
Week 4	2-2½ miles	13-25 min./mile
Week 5	2½-3 miles	13-20 min./mile
Week 6	2½-3 miles	13-20 min./mile
Week 7	3-4 miles	13-20 min./mile
Week 8	3-4 miles	13-20 min./mile
Week 9	4-5 miles	13-20 min./mile
Week 10	4-5 miles	13-20 min./mile
Week 11	5-6 miles	13-20 min./mile
Week 12	5-6 miles	13-20 min./mile

Walking

A brisk walk lasting 30 to 60 minutes most days of the week can provide many of the benefits of aerobic exercise. Even walking at a slow pace can lower your risk of heart disease, although faster, farther and more frequent walking offers even greater health benefits. Plus, walking is easy to do.

Jogging

Like walking, jogging is an excellent form of aerobic exercise. And like walking, jogging doesn't have to be strenuous to have a positive effect. Even when done at low intensity, jogging is a good way to increase cardiovascular fitness.

Jogging for 30 minutes three times a week can help you achieve cardiovascular fitness, but it won't prepare you to complete a marathon. If your goal is to run a marathon, a more vigorous, structured training program is necessary.

Hiking

Hiking can be as intense a workout as you want it to be. A beginner can stick to short, level trails; an advanced hiker can trek through miles of hilly terrain. Hiking helps to increase your endurance and muscle strength. Depending on your route, it works different muscles than does walking.

Bicycling

Bicycling revs up your cardiovascular fitness while strengthening your leg muscles. It offers a great deal of freedom, plus a welcome change of scenery from one session to the next, and it's a good low-impact activity.

Like traditional bikes, a stationary bike also provides aerobic exercise. Stationary bikes can be upright or reclining (recumbent). One type of stationary bike isn't inherently better than another, although recumbent bikes may be more comfortable for people with back or neck pain.

Water exercise

If you want a low-impact activity that exercises your entire body, swimming may be right for you. Swimming is often recommended for people with muscle and joint problems. If lap swimming isn't your style, you might consider taking

GETTING STARTED ON A JOGGING PROGRAM

Many people enjoy the challenge of training for local fun runs and road races, while others enjoy the benefits of jogging in weight management.

The key is to start slowly. Advance one step in this starter program every 2 to 7 days, as you feel able. If you're in step 1, jog for one minute, then walk for one minute. Repeat this until you've jogged and walked for a total of 24 minutes (12 repetitions). When you're comfortable with this portion of the program, move up to step 2. Continue moving up in steps as you're able. By step 10, you'll be able to jog through an entire workout.

The whole program looks like this:

	Time		Repetitions		Total time
	Jog	Walk	Jog	Walk	
Step 1	1 min.	1 min.	12	12	24 min.
Step 2	2 min.	1 min.	8	8	24 min.
Step 3	3 min.	1 min.	6	6	24 min.
Step 4	4 min.	1 min.	5	5	25 min.
Step 5	5 min.	1 min.	4	4	24 min.
Step 6	7 min.	1 min.	3	2	23 min.
Step 7	10 min.	1 min.	2	2	22 min.
Step 8	12 min.	1 min.	2	1	25 min.
Step 9	15 min.	1 min.	2	1	31 min.
Step 10	20 min.	—	1	—	20 min.
Step 11	25 min.	—	1	—	25 min.
Step 12	30 min.	—	1	—	30 min.

part in a water aerobics class or just walking in the pool.

The benefits of water exercises are that they can work all of your muscles and they're generally easy on your joints. This is because the buoyancy of water reduces pressure on your joints. Water exercises, however, aren't the best method for weight loss. If weight loss is one of your goals, you might consider supplementing your water workout with other forms of exercise, such as bicycling or walking.

Aerobic dance and stepping

Low-impact aerobic dance exercises the whole body while you move to music. Classes are usually offered for a variety of levels, although at any time you can alter your movements to whatever intensity you choose. Of course, the intensity will determine the benefits you derive.

Like aerobic dancing, stepping is a popular exercise for people of all abilities. Using a short, stable platform-type

WARMING UP AND COOLING DOWN

Whatever your activity, make sure to warm up before exercise and cool down afterward. Warming up and cooling down help reduce the risk of injuries and muscle damage.

A warmup prepares the body for exercise. It gradually revs up your cardiovascular system, increases blood flow to your muscles and raises your body temperature. Start your workout with a few minutes of low-intensity, whole-body exercise, such as walking or pedaling on a stationary bike.

Immediately after your workout, take time to cool down. This gradually brings down the temperature of your muscle tissue and may help reduce muscle injury, stiffness and soreness. Mild activity after exercise also prevents blood from pooling in your legs. Cooling down is similar to warming up. After your workout, walk or continue your activity at a low intensity for 5 to 10 minutes.

HOW MANY CALORIES DOES IT BURN?

Burning about 1,000 calories a week with exercise significantly improves your overall health. This chart shows the estimated calories used while performing various activities for one hour. The figures represent a moderately intense level of exercise. The more you weigh, the more calories you use. Note that these figures are estimates — actual calories used vary from person to person.

Calories used

Activity (1 hour duration)	160 lb. person	200 lb. person	240 lb. person
Aerobics, low-impact	365	455	545
Aerobics, water	402	501	600
Bicycling, less than 10 mph	292	364	436
Bowling	219	273	327
Dancing, ballroom	219	273	327
Elliptical trainer, moderate effort	365	455	545
Golfing, carrying clubs	314	391	469
Hiking	438	546	654
Ice skating	511	637	763
Jogging, 5 mph	606	755	905
Racquetball, casual	511	637	763
Resistance (weight) training	365	455	545
Rowing, stationary	438	546	654
Running, 8 mph	861	1,074	1,286
Skiing, cross-country	496	619	741
Skiing, downhill	314	391	469
Softball or baseball	365	455	545
Stair treadmill	657	819	981
Swimming, laps, light or moderate	423	528	632
Tennis, singles	584	728	872
Volleyball	292	364	436
Walking, 2 mph	204	255	305
Walking, 3½ mph	314	391	469
Yoga, hatha	183	228	273

Adapted from B. E. Ainsworth et al., *Medicine and Science in Sports and Exercise* 43 (2011): 8.

bench, exercisers step up and down to music during each session. Low-impact stepping can be a fun, motivating way to exercise — increasing your endurance and lower-body muscle strength.

RESISTANCE TRAINING

When it comes to overall fitness, investing in a set of weights, resistance bands or other related equipment may pay dividends just as great as those gained with a pair of walking shoes. The more fit your muscles are, the easier your daily tasks become, whether they include lifting a load of wet laundry or shoveling snow.

Resistance training, also known as strength training, involves the use of free weights, your own body weight, resistance bands or tubing, or a weight (resistance) machine to increase muscle strength and endurance. You can choose one method or combine them for greater variety.

Adults of all ages can benefit from regular resistance training. If you're inactive, you can lose up to 10% of your lean muscle mass each decade after age 30. Resistance training can help preserve and enhance your muscle mass, which becomes important with age.

Resistance training can help you:
- Increase the strength of your muscles, help protect your joints and decrease your risk of injury. Injury from falls is a common problem as we get older.
- Increase the density of your bones, reducing the risk of osteoporosis. If you already have osteoporosis, strength training can lessen the condition's impact.
- Achieve better balance, coordination and agility.
- Strengthen muscles in your abdomen and lumbar region, reducing chronic low-back pain.

You don't need to spend 90 minutes a day lifting weights to benefit from strength training. In fact, it's better that you not lift weights every day. Strength training sessions lasting 20 to 30 minutes and done just two or three times a week are sufficient for most people and can result in significant, noticeable improvements. Another option, if you use resistance bands, is to perform resistance exercises daily but alternate the muscle groups involved (see "Have a plan" on the next page).

Free weights

Free weights refers to items such as barbells and dumbbells. These are the basic tools of strength training. Plastic soft drink bottles filled with water or sand may also work for you.

When using weights, your movements should be slow and deliberate. If you experience pain in any of your joints when using weights, reduce the amount of weight or switch to a different exercise. Just one set of 12 repetitions twice a week produces 85% of the total benefit gained from use of free weights.

Resistance machines and home gyms

These machines typically work different parts of your body with controlled

---

HAVE A PLAN

It's important not to exercise the same muscles two days in a row. You want to rest at least one full day between exercising each muscle group. Consider developing a plan for working specific muscle groups on given days. For example, on Mondays and Thursdays you work your chest, shoulders, quadriceps and triceps — those muscles that push. On Tuesdays and Fridays you can work your back, hamstrings and biceps — the muscles that pull.

To begin, select a weight that you can lift comfortably 15 to 20 times. A weight that fatigues your muscles after 12 repetitions is an ideal stimulus for muscle strength and tone. Repetitions refer to the number of times you lift the weight or, if you're using a weight machine, push against the resistance. If you're a beginner, you may discover that you're able to lift only one or two pounds or less. That's OK. Once your muscles, tendons and ligaments grow accustomed to strength exercises, you'll be surprised at how you progress.

Don't rush your movements. Follow proper technique and lift or push the weight as you count slowly to three. Hold the position for one second, then lower the weight as you slowly count to three. Your movements should be unhurried and controlled.

weights and resistance. Some have stacked weights, others have bendable plastic pieces, and still others have hydraulic components. Each of these devices works by providing resistance to motion in some way.

Proper instruction is essential for safe use. Ask an individual trained in exercise techniques how to use the equipment to make sure you're getting the maximum benefit. Resistance machines often must be adjusted to your height and arm and leg lengths in order to ensure proper form during exercise.

Resistance bands or tubing

These elastic-like cords, tubing or flat bands offer progressively increasing resistance when you pull on them. They come in different tensions to fit a range of abilities and are usually color-coded. Resistance bands are portable and an inexpensive alternative to a home gym.

CORE STABILITY TRAINING

Core stability training is a type of strength training. It works the muscles

YOU CAN BE STRONG AT ANY AGE

It wasn't that long ago that scientists believed that a substantial loss of strength was an inevitable part of aging. After all, some decrease in muscle mass is a normal part of getting older. It's now clear that if you're dedicated to maintaining your strength, you can make great strides in doing so as you age.

Studies show that strength can be maintained and perhaps increased at any age — even in your 80s and beyond. The key is to dedicate yourself to a regular and progressive program of resistance (strength) exercises.

In one study, people in their late 80s and early 90s performed regular strength-training exercises over a 12-week period. The results showed an average increase of 175% in the strength of the participants' upper thigh muscles (quadriceps). Participants also improved their balance and found climbing stairs easier.

in the midsection of your body. Additional benefits of core stability training include increased flexibility and better balance.

The core of your body — the area around your trunk — is where your center of gravity is located. Your core is your body's foundation, linking your upper body and lower body. When you have good core stability, the muscles in your abdomen, pelvis, lower back and hips work together, stabilizing the rest of your body and providing support to your spine.

Developing a strong, solid core gives you increased balance. A strong core can help prevent poor posture and low-back pain. For many people, the prevention of low-back pain is a compelling argument for exercising core muscles. Regular aerobic and strength training exercises often don't build core strength because most of them focus on arm and leg strength.

Essentially any exercise that uses the trunk of your body without support is a core exercise. For example, a pushup stresses your core more than does a bench press, during which the bench is supporting your trunk. As a result, nearly any exercise can be modified to increase your core activity.

It's a good idea to get some personal instruction as you begin a core training program, because pinpointing your core muscles takes some practice. Taking a class with a certified fitness instructor can help you make sure you're using the correct muscles. Whichever core exercises you choose, aim to do them three times a week or every other day.

Core stability exercises include floor exercises, workouts using a fitness ball, and Pilates.

Floor exercises

Perhaps the two most important deep core muscles are your transversus abdominis, located deep in a hooplike ring around your abdomen, and your multifidus, found in your back. You can find and strengthen these key muscles with specific exercises that require nothing but your body and the floor.

Fitness ball workouts

Fitness balls, which look like large, sturdy beach balls, can be used to work the deep core muscles of your abdomen and back. If you're stocking a home gym, fitness balls are a versatile investment. They're also called stability balls, physioballs or Swiss balls — because they were first used in Switzerland many years ago to help rehabilitate people with stroke-related disabilities.

These balls not only work the trunk in almost every exercise they're designed for, but also help with balance and flexibility exercises. When strengthening your core with a fitness ball, you want to create a balance between your abdominal muscles and your back muscles by doing exercises that work each equally. This is important because if there's imbalance in your abdomen or your back muscles, pain and poor posture can result.

Pilates

Pilates is a low-impact fitness technique developed in the 1920s by Joseph Pilates. Designed specifically to strengthen the body's core muscles by developing pelvic stability and abdominal control, Pilates exercises also help improve flexibility, joint mobility and strength. They can help you develop long, strong muscles, maintain a strong back and improve your posture.

Many Pilates exercises are done with special machines. The earliest Pilates machine, known as the Reformer, was a wooden device outfitted with cables, pulleys, springs and sliding boards.

Although machines are still used, many Pilates programs offer floor-work classes as well, designed to stabilize and strengthen the core back and abdominal muscles.

Instead of emphasizing quantity, Pilates focuses on quality, meaning that exercisers do very few, but extremely precise, repetitions. Exercises can be adapted according to a person's own flexibility and strength abilities. It may be a good idea to review the Pilates approach before committing to a class.

FLEXIBILITY EXERCISES

When you hear the words *flexible* and *agile*, you may think of Olympic gymnasts or world-class ballerinas. But the truth is that everyone is flexible to some degree, and almost anyone can acquire greater flexibility. Flexibility is the ability to move your joints through their full range of motion.

Like many other indicators of fitness, your flexibility may diminish as you get older. But like other effects of aging and inactivity, flexibility can be regained and maintained.

Increased flexibility, which is achieved by regularly stretching muscles, will help improve your daily activites of living. Routine tasks are easier and less tiring when your muscles and joints have good flexibility. Flexibility exercises also help improve posture and coordination.

A regular stretching program is the most common way to increase your flexibility, but other activities such as swimming, yoga and tai chi are also effective for improving flexibility.

Stretching

Stretching is a common way to gain range of motion in a joint, and nearly anyone can do it. It's truly one of the easiest exercises to work into your routine.

A good rule of thumb is to spend 5 to 10 minutes stretching before your workouts (after a short five-minute warmup) and another 5 to 10 minutes afterward. In addition to stretching before and after aerobic and strength training, you may want to adopt a stretching program. If

THE RIGHT WAY TO STRETCH

Before stretching, take a few minutes to warm your muscles. Stretching muscles when they're cold increases your risk of injury, including pulled muscles. Warm up by doing a low-intensity exercise, such as walking while gently swinging your arms, for at least five minutes.

With today's busy schedules and hectic demands, if you have time to stretch only once, do it after you exercise. This is when blood flow to your muscles is increased, and the tissues are more flexible.

Stretching techniques are fairly simple and easy to learn. Here are some guidelines to consider:
• Hold your stretches for at least 30 seconds, and up to a minute for a really tight muscle or problem area. That can seem like a long time, so use a watch or count out loud to make sure you're holding your stretches long enough.

you can, try to stretch three days a week. Each day focus on different muscle groups. One day you might focus on your neck and shoulders, another day on your hips and lower back, and another day on your calves and thighs.

Also stretch any muscles and joints that you routinely use. If you frequently play tennis or golf, for example, working in extra shoulder stretches loosens the muscles around your shoulder joint, making it feel less tight and more ready for action.

Yoga

Yoga, which combines deep breathing, movement and postures, can reduce anxiety, strengthen muscles, lower blood pressure and help your heart work more efficiently.

Yoga's techniques for stretching and strengthening the body can be practiced by people of all ages. However, adults with osteoporosis, older adults or those with stiff joints may have to eliminate and adapt some of the traditional poses.

- When you begin a stretch, spend the first 15 seconds in an easy stretch. Stretch just until you feel a mild tension, then relax as you hold the stretch. The tension should be comfortable, not painful.
- Once you've completed the easy stretch, stretch just a fraction of an inch farther until you again feel mild tension. Hold it for 15 seconds. Again, you should feel tension, but not pain.
- Relax and breathe freely while you're stretching. Try not to hold your breath. If you're bending forward to do a stretch, exhale as you bend forward and then breathe slowly as you hold the stretch.
- Avoid bouncing. This can cause small tears in muscle, which leave scar tissue as the muscle heals. The scar tightens the muscle further, making you even less flexible and more prone to pain.
- Avoid locking your joints. Bend your joints slightly while stretching.

If you've had joint replacement surgery, especially hip replacement, some yoga positions may put you at risk of injury and joint dislocation. If you've had such surgery, be sure to talk with your doctor before starting yoga.

Yoga can be as vigorous or as gentle as you choose. Different styles appeal to different people, depending on their goals and ability levels. Some styles offer gentle movements combined with deep breathing, while others are fast paced or are practiced in rooms heated to more than 100 F, known as hot yoga. Before joining a class, test it out first to make sure it fits your skill level and preferences.

Feldenkrais Method

The Feldenkrais Method uses gentle movements to develop increased flexibility and coordination. Though similar to yoga, the Feldenkrais Method doesn't strive for correct positions but instead aims for more dexterous, painless and efficient body movements.

The goal is to create an awareness and quality of movement through your body feedback rather than through pre-defined postures. These techniques often are used in physical and occupational therapies.

BALANCE EXERCISES

Balance is the ability to control your center of gravity over your base of support. It's related to your strength, inner ear balance center (vestibular system), vision and sensory input from your feet as well as your muscles and tendons. The balance required to complete daily tasks is often taken for granted in adulthood, but the truth is that if you don't use your balancing skills, you may lose them.

Balance exercises — activities you do to hone your balance and coordination skills — are beneficial for all people, but especially for older adults. Balance exercises can help prevent falls, improve your coordination, make you more confident about your stability and boost your feelings of security. When combined with strength training, balance exercises help build muscle around your joints, making the joints more stable so that you feel steadier on your feet. People who do balance exercises have greater mobility as they age.

Almost any activity that keeps you on your feet and moving is helpful in maintaining good balance. Basic exercises that get your legs and arms moving at the same time can help you maintain your balance, in addition to stimulating the muscle and nerve communication that increases your coordination.

Tai chi

This ancient form of martial arts involves gentle, circular movements combined with deep breathing. Tai chi helps improve balance, strength and flexibility and reduces stress. Tai chi may also help you build stamina and experience greater relaxation.

Tai chi consists of a series of graceful movements that improve stance and coordination. You learn how to turn your body more slowly and gain more confidence in your movements. Each of these benefits can result in better balance.

Health clubs and community centers frequently offer classes with experienced instructors. An experienced instructor is your best bet for reaping all the benefits of tai chi. Whether you take a class, rent a video or refer to a book, look for instruction that's geared to your age group or activity level.

Individual exercises

Individual exercises used to improve balance include standing on one leg,

using a weight in only one hand or standing on a pillow or foam pad while performing an exercise. For each of the variations, if you're worried about losing your balance, make sure someone is nearby to help you, or position yourself to hold on to a railing or stable surface.

EXERCISE GUIDE

Your health care team or a physical or exercise therapist can help identify the best exercises for you based on your individual health and fitness goals. The exercises that follow in this chapter are commonly recommended to build strength, including core strength, and to promote balance and improve flexibility.

You may benefit by including some or all of them in your regular activity routine. It's not necessary to do the exercises every day or to do all of them on the same day. Aim to perform the exercises a couple of times a week, spreading them out over the week. Also, don't perform any exercises that could cause you injury or place you at risk of a fall.

Getting and staying motivated

Remember that physical fitness is a journey, not a destination. Fitness is not a goal you simply achieve one day and then are done with. It's something you strive for, for the rest of your life.

As with any journey, you may encounter some roadblocks and setbacks. For some people, getting started is the hardest step. Others begin with tremendous enthusiasm and go at it so vigorously that they get hurt and stop.

To have the best chance of success — a lifelong commitment to physical activity — you need to get and stay motivated. Exercise has to be as natural and ingrained a habit as is brushing your teeth or taking a shower.

With the right frame of mind, anyone can get and stay motivated to exercise. People who are self-motivated are more likely to stick with an exercise program than those who rely solely on external forms of motivation. If your motivation is internally based, you're doing the activity for yourself — because you enjoy it, because you want to look or feel better, because you want to become healthier or because you've been diagnosed with a health condition, such as heart disease, diabetes or cancer.

External motivation, in contrast, comes from outside — you're exercising to please someone else or to reach a particular goal, such as a 10-pound weight loss, or a reward, such as new clothes. You're more focused on the outcome than the process.

The bottom line is that you'll be more motivated if you can embrace the activity as something you want to do for yourself over the long term.

The payoff

Longevity is affected by some things you simply cannot control, such as your genes. But of those factors that you can control, being physically active — moving more and sitting less — is one of the most important steps that you can take to both extend and improve the quality of your life.

Regardless of your age, the time you invest now in becoming more physically active and staying fit will pay off in the years to come. And before you know it, you'll have a well-developed, personalized plan that makes exercise a regular part of your life.

You don't have to come up with a perfect plan, but adopt a fitness routine that you can enjoy for life. In addition to aerobic activities, include strength, flexibility and balance exercises.

Squats

Stand with a sturdy chair behind you. Hold on to a counter for support. Breathe out as you squat down as far as you can comfortably go, keeping knees in line with your toes. Hold the position for five seconds. Inhale as you return to standing. Relax and repeat. As you build strength, hold the squat for longer or squat down farther.

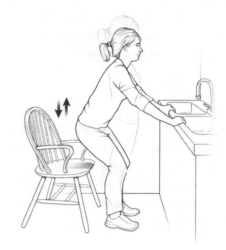

Sit-to-stand

Sit in a sturdy chair with arms. Keeping your spine straight, raise yourself up off the chair without using your arms or hands to assist you. Keep your knees over your toes during the motion. Relax and repeat. If your legs are weak, you may need to push your body up using your arms or hands to assist you. Relax and repeat.

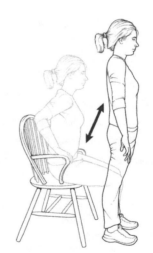

Biceps strengthening

Sit in a sturdy chair with a length of resistance tubing. Grasp one end of the tubing in each hand and place your hands on your knees, with palms up and arms straight. Pull upward with one arm, as shown. Slowly return to the starting position and repeat with the other arm.

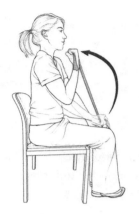

Triceps strengthening

Grasp one end of the resistance tubing in each hand and hold both hands at shoulder height, with thumbs up and elbows bent. Straighten one arm toward your knee, keeping your elbow at your side. Slowly return to the starting position and repeat with the other arm.

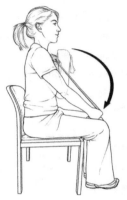

Toe lift

Stand with your feet as wide as your hips. Hold on to a counter for support. Keeping your heels firmly planted, lift your toes as high as you can. Lower your toes and repeat.

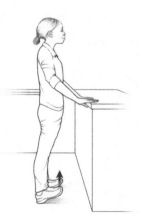

Heel lift

Stand with your feet as wide as your hips. Hold on to a counter for support. Keeping your toes firmly planted, lift your heels as high as you can. Lower your heels and repeat.

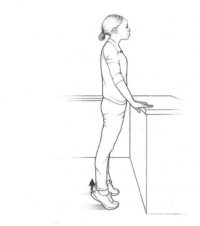

Pelvic tilt

Lie on a firm, flat surface with your knees bent. Place your hands across your chest. The natural curves of the spine in your neck and lower back may not be touching the underlying surface. Tighten your abdominal muscles to flatten the small of your back against the surface. Release tension in your abdominal muscles to arch the small of your back (lower right). Slowly return to the starting position. Relax and repeat.

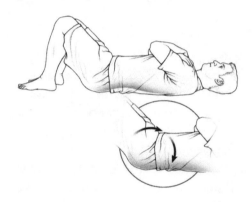

Lower back extension

Lie facedown, placing your hands alongside your chest. Relax in this position briefly. Use your arms to lift your upper body until your arms are straight. Lift only as high as is comfortable. Look straight ahead and relax your stomach and lower back. Stay in this position briefly and then lower your body to the surface. Relax and repeat.

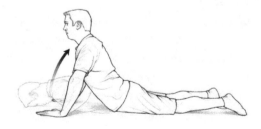

Modified plank

Lie on your stomach with your knees hip-width apart. Bend your elbows so that your forearms rest on the floor. Slowly raise your body, keeping your abdominal muscles tight, your elbows under your shoulders, your head in line with your spine and your knees on the floor. Hold the position for a few seconds and slowly return to the starting position. Relax and repeat. If you're able, you can perform this exercise lifting your knees and keeping only your toes and forearms on the floor.

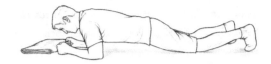

Bridge

Lie on your back with your knees bent and your feet flat on the surface. Place your arms out to your sides for balance. Slowly lift your hips without arching your back, keeping your hips level. Squeeze your buttocks muscles together. Hold briefly and slowly return to the starting position. Relax and repeat.

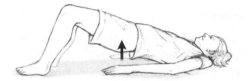

Cat stretch

Get on your hands and knees. Arch your back away from the floor and then let it sag toward the floor. Focus on your mid to lower back, where the motion should be taking place. Don't arch your head backward too far. Relax and repeat.

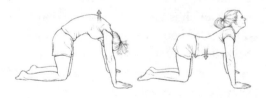

Lower back stretches

Lie on your back, with your knees bent and feet on the floor. Keeping your lower back on the floor, lift your right knee and hug it toward your chest, using your hands (top). Hold this position for a few deep breaths. Repeat with the left knee. Then hug both knees (bottom). If knee pain is aggravated by this exercise, place your hands behind the knee joints when pulling your knees toward your chest.

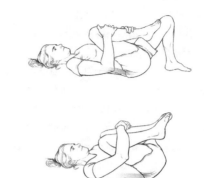

Lumbar rotation

Lie on your back, with knees bent and feet on the floor. Place your hands behind your head with your elbows out. Gently roll your knees to the left, all the way to the floor if you can. Hold this position for a few deep breaths. Return to the starting position. Then roll to the right. Repeat.

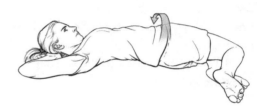

Sitting lumbar stretch

Sit in a chair. Bring your chin toward your chest and let your hands drop toward the floor. Slowly bend forward until you feel a stretch in your lower back. Hold the position briefly and return to a sitting position.

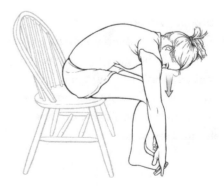

Neck stretches

Tilt your chin forward and down to your chest, then tilt your chin back and upward (left illustrations). Next, tilt your ear toward one shoulder and then the other, without raising your shoulders (upper right illustration). Finally, turn your face to the left, keeping your neck, shoulders and spine straight, then turn your face to the right (lower right illustration).

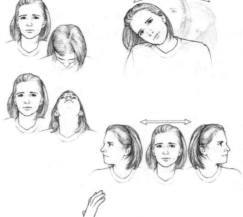

Overhead arm raise

Stand with your arms straight out at chest height. Gently raise your arms over your head. Lower them back to the starting position. Relax and repeat.

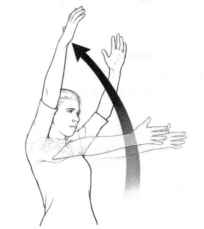

Overhead shoulder stretch

Place one arm behind your head. Using your other hand, grasp the overhead arm just above the elbow and gently pull the elbow downward until you feel a gentle stretch in your shoulder. Hold briefly. Relax and switch arms.

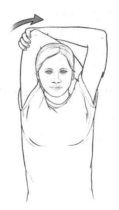

Horizontal shoulder rotation

Keeping your back straight, use the hand of one arm to cradle the elbow of the opposite arm. Pull the arm being cradled across your chest until you feel a gentle stretch in the shoulder. Hold briefly. Relax and switch arms.

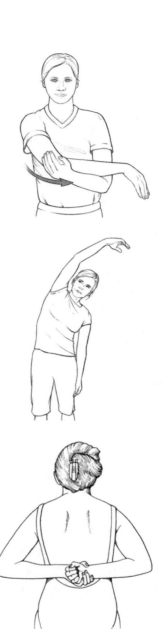

Side bend

Stand facing forward with your feet comfortably apart. Lean to one side as you bring the opposite arm up over your head. Let your other arm hang to your side. Hold the position briefly. Relax and switch arms.

Behind-the-back stretch

Grasp one wrist behind your back. Gently pull your arm up until you feel a stretch in your shoulders. Relax and repeat. Switch arms.

Shoulder-blade squeeze

Raise your hands behind your head with your arms out to the side. Pinch your shoulder blades together by moving your elbows back. Hold briefly. Relax and repeat.

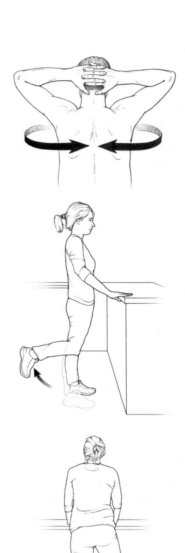

Knee bend

Stand with your feet as wide as your hips. You may hold on to a counter for support. Slowly bend one knee, bringing your heel up toward your buttocks, and hold for a few seconds. Return to the starting position and repeat with the other knee. To help improve balance, stand in place for progressively longer periods of time with your knee bent.

Hip swing

Stand with your feet shoulder-width apart. You may hold on to a counter for support. Slowly swing one foot off the floor to the side, as far as you can, and hold. Keep your spine neutral and do not allow it to bend, twist or rotate during the hip-swing motion. Return to the starting position and repeat with the other foot. To work on balance, remove one hand from the counter.

Calf stretch

Stand with your hands pressing against a wall. Bring one leg back, keeping the knee straight and your foot flat on the floor. Lean on your front, slightly bent leg until you feel a stretch in the calf of your back leg and hold for a few seconds. Return to the starting position and repeat with your other leg.

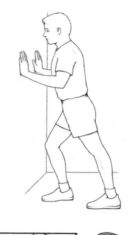

Thigh stretch

Stand and place one hand on a wall or a sturdy piece of furniture. With your other hand, grab your ankle. Slowly pull the bent leg toward your buttock until you feel a moderate stretch in the muscles in the front of your thigh. Hold briefly and return to the starting position. Switch arms and repeat with the other leg. When doing this exercise, if you cannot reach your ankle, grab the hem of your pants.

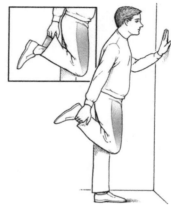

Standing march

Stand between a counter and a sturdy chair. Hold on to the counter and chair for support, if needed. Keep your spine straight and slowly march in place, lifting your feet as high as you can.

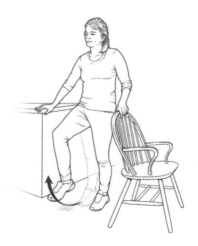

Single leg stand

Stand with both feet on the floor and your arms held out or by your sides. If you're concerned you could fall, hold on to a chair or counter with one arm. Bending at the knee, lift one leg and hold the position for a few seconds. Place your lifted leg back on the floor, relax and repeat. Switch to the other leg.

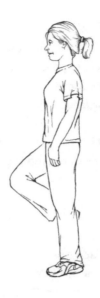

15

Eating well to live well

Diet is the top risk factor for disease and early death worldwide. Heart disease is our No. 1 killer, and what we put in our mouths is the biggest driving force behind it. Close behind is cancer, and at least a dozen cancers are linked to weight and obesity. Diet also has a profound effect on aging, and a poor diet increases the risk of other diseases such as diabetes.

A study published in the journal *The Lancet* found that annually, about 11 million deaths worldwide are linked to poor diets. And, unlike many other risk factors, a bad diet affects all ages, male and female, from all walks of life.

Today we have more food available than ever before. And yet food is proving to be our undoing. Our diets are out of balance. We're not eating enough of the foods that nourish us — fruits, vegetables, legumes, nuts and whole grains, for example. And we're consuming too much of the foods that, in excess, put us in danger — a lot of meat, sugar, salt and fat.

The evidence is overwhelmingly clear that good food is crucial to good health.

The decisions you make each day regarding what you eat affect how well you'll live now and in years ahead. That's because you really are what you eat!

Your health is greatly influenced by the interaction of nutrients and genes — a continual interplay in which certain foods enhance the action of protective (or harmful) genes, while other foods try to suppress them. People who regularly enjoy meals made with a variety of healthy ingredients generally are at less risk of developing many diseases.

The bottom line: If you want to live well, you have to eat well.

WHAT'S A HEALTHY DIET?

To eat healthy, it's not necessary to follow a specialized diet, but it is important to eat a balanced diet. Eating well means enjoying great taste as well as great nutrition.

The pages that follow contain the latest information about how the food you eat can help keep you healthy. By learning more about how your body uses the different nutrients found in food, you'll better understand how what you eat everyday affects how you function today and in years to come.

While we know that diet has a powerful effect on health, nutrition can be a complicated topic. It's not always easy to tease out specific associations between health benefits and certain foods. But what research has found, more often than not, is that certain patterns of eating tend to be associated with greater health. For example, plant-based diets along with lean proteins seem to have the greatest benefit in terms of preventing common chronic diseases such as heart disease, cancer and dementia.

The Mediterranean diet, which embraces a plant-based approach, is one such diet. The Mayo Clinic diet, which is similar in many ways to the Mediterranean diet, is another. One of the main benefits of both diet plans is their anti-inflammatory properties — the way they help reduce chronic low-grade inflammation, a condition that underlies so many chronic diseases.

The focus on fruits, vegetables and whole grains inherent in both diets increases consumption of soluble fiber, which scores high marks for its anti-inflammatory properties. Healthy sources of fat, such as olive oil, increase intake of monounsaturated fats, which also have anti-inflammatory properties. Fish, another staple in both diets, is rich in omega-3 fatty acids, a type of

THE MAYO CLINIC HEALTHY WEIGHT PYRAMID

The Mayo Clinic diet is based on the Mayo Clinic Healthy Weight Pyramid, which includes six sections, representing six food groups. Foods are grouped according to common health benefits that they share and their levels of energy density. All foods contain a certain number of calories (energy) within a given amount (volume). Some foods contain many calories in just a small portion, such as fats. They're described as high in energy density. Foods with fewer calories in a larger volume, such as vegetables and fruits, are low in energy density.

Foods high in energy density are at the top of the pyramid — you want to eat less of these. Those low in energy density are at the bottom of the pyramid — you want to eat more of these. Foods low in energy density are generally healthier, and you get a lot more food for the calories.

The Mayo Clinic Healthy Weight Pyramid was developed not only to help people eat more nutritiously but also to help individuals who are overweight achieve a weight that's healthier.

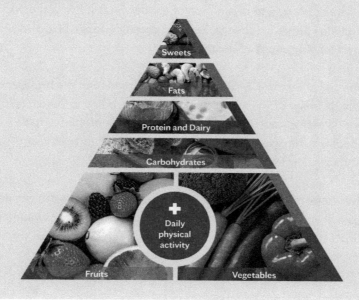

polyunsaturated fat also thought to curb inflammation.

Anti-inflammatory properties of both dietary approaches appear to directly correlate with why they decrease the risk of death from heart disease, stroke and cancer, as well as lower the risk of developing diabetes, Alzheimer's disease, arthritis, Parkinson's disease and other illnesses. In addition, vegetables, fruits and whole grains are endowed

FIBER, HEALTH AND MORTALITY

Hundreds of thousands of years ago, our fiber intake was very high due to the foraging practices of our ancestors. Today, most people don't get enough. Current guidelines recommend a daily fiber intake of 14 grams for every 1,000 calories consumed — or about 25 grams a day for women, 38 grams for men. But average fiber consumption among Americans is only 17 grams a day.

This is problematic because it means that most Americans are missing out on all of fiber's benefits. Fiber lowers blood pressure, blood sugar levels and blood cholesterol, and it's linked to prevention of cancer. Plus, it fills you up on fewer calories and helps prevent constipation. Not getting enough fiber has been shown to be a leading cause of death.

Fiber works in a variety of ways. It reduces inflammation in the body, and it improves the diversity of the gut microbiome — the healthy, beneficial bacteria living in your digestive tract. In your gut, fiber acts as a prebiotic, food for the beneficial bacteria that live there. Fiber also helps your body efficiently use nutrients and calories, and it boosts your immune system.

As part of your efforts to improve your diet, make sure that you're getting enough fiber. Foods high in fiber include citrus fruits, apples, pears, most vegetables, legumes (dried beans and peas), oatmeal and oat bran, wheat bran, and whole-grain breads, pasta and cereals. See the chart on page 113.

with many nutrients and health-enhancing compounds called phytochemicals, which experts believe work together to fight disease.

Vegetables

It's hardly news that vegetables are good for you. The real news is why. Each decade we're learning more about how fresh produce, such as vegetables and fruits, can supply us with vital substances that ward off many illnesses and diseases.

Strong evidence is stacking up that people who eat generous helpings of a variety of vegetables run a lower risk of developing heart disease, a leading killer of American adults. In addition, researchers have identified substances in vegetables called phytochemicals that appear to offer some protection against cancer.

Most vegetables are loaded with the antioxidants beta carotene and vitamin C. Antioxidants can be important because these substances play a role in inhibiting molecules called oxygen-free radicals, which can damage healthy cells in the body. Vegetables are also key sources of essential vitamins and minerals, including folate, potassium,

magnesium and selenium. Many are rich in health-enhancing fiber, and some even have calcium. Vegetables contain no cholesterol, and they're naturally low in fat and calories.

Fruits

Fruits, like many vegetables, have an abundance of vitamins, minerals and fiber, not to mention a long list of healthy antioxidants, including vitamin C. Some fruits, as well as vegetables, contain the antioxidants lutein and zeaxanthin, which may guard against certain conditions related to aging, such as macular degeneration, a disease that affects vision.

Researchers have discovered that many fruits, as well as vegetables, contain generous amounts of flavonoids. These are compounds extracted from plants that fight off harmful molecules that cause oxidative stress, thereby reducing your risk of cancer and heart disease. Oranges and avocados, for instance, are rich in a flavonoid compound called beta-sitosterol, which is believed to help lower blood cholesterol.

As with vegetables, because different fruits provide different nutrients, variety is important.

Carbohydrates

Envision every kind of food containing carbohydrates laid out in a line. At one end are whole wheat, oats and brown rice. In the middle sit white bread, white rice, potatoes and pasta. And at the far end are cookies, candies and soft drinks. The foods in this spectrum incorporate all three kinds of carbohydrates: fiber, starch and sugar.

It's not hard to determine the healthy and unhealthy ends — unrefined whole grains on one end and refined sugar on the other. The foods in the middle — rice, pasta, bread and potatoes — are all nutritious, but can lose some of their health benefits depending on how they're processed and prepared.

Whole grains are the types of carbohydrates that you should eat the most of. Some are rich in vitamin E, an antioxidant with many health benefits. Others contain lignans, estrogen-like substances that may help protect against some forms of cancer. All contain fiber that's good for digestive health.

Protein and dairy

Protein is essential to human life. But it's not necessary or even desirable to eat meat every day to get needed protein. Other foods that provide protein include low-fat dairy products, seafood and many plant foods. Legumes — namely beans, lentils and peas — are excellent sources of protein. That's because they have no cholesterol and very little fat. In addition, the fiber in beans helps lower LDL blood cholesterol, and the minerals they contain help control blood pressure.

It's also important that you include fish and shellfish in your diet. Not only do they provide protein, but some supply omega-3 fatty acids. Omega-3 fats help lower triglycerides, fat particles in the blood that appear to raise heart disease risk. Omega-3s may also improve immune function and help regulate blood pressure. Research suggests that most people would benefit from eating at least two servings of fish a week.

Fats

Not all fat is bad for you. Some kinds are actually beneficial. Therefore, it's important that you include some fat in your diet. The keys are not to eat too much and to eat the right kinds.

High-fat plant foods, such as avocados, olives, seeds and nuts, and some cooking oils, such as canola and olive, are good for you. Nuts, for instance, contain monounsaturated fat, which helps keep harmful deposits from accumulating in blood vessels and lowers your heart attack risk. They also provide other key nutrients.

But even though nuts, vegetable oils and avocados may be beneficial, use them in moderation. A tablespoon of peanut butter weighs in at nearly 100 calories and a tablespoon of olive oil at 140. An avocado contains between 200 and 300 calories, depending on size.

In other words, the goal is to eat enough of these foods to gain their health benefits but not so much that you consume too many calories. Most nutrition experts recommend no more than 3 to 5 servings daily.

Sweets

Foods in the sweets group include candies, cookies and other desserts. And don't forget the sugar you may add to your cereal, coffee or other beverages. Sweets are high in energy density and calories, and they offer little to nothing in terms of nutrition. You want to limit the amount of sweets you eat, which also includes alcohol.

LOVABLE LEGUMES

The term *legume* refers to a large family of plants, including beans, lentils and peas, whose seeds develop inside pods and are usually dried for ease of storage.

Legumes are low in fat and high in fiber, protein, folate, potassium, iron, magnesium and phytochemicals. The fiber in legumes is mostly soluble, which studies show may help lower cholesterol and help regulate blood sugar levels. In addition, legumes — which include soybeans, peanuts, lima beans, chickpeas, black-eyed peas, split peas and lentils — are versatile and inexpensive. They're a healthy substitute for meat, which has more fat and cholesterol. If you use canned legumes, rinse them well to eliminate salt that may have been added during processing.

SHAKING THE SALT HABIT

Salt, also known as sodium chloride, is about 40% sodium and 60% chloride. It flavors food and is used as a binder and stabilizer. It's also a food preservative because bacteria can't thrive amid a high amount of salt. The human body requires a small amount of sodium to conduct nerve impulses, contract and relax muscles, and maintain the proper balance of water and minerals. Too much sodium in your diet can lead to high blood pressure and other diseases. It may also cause calcium loss.

When your sodium levels are low, your kidneys essentially hold on to the sodium. When sodium levels are high, your kidneys excrete the excess in urine. When your kidneys can't eliminate sodium, it starts to accumulate in your blood. Because sodium attracts and holds water, your blood volume increases. Increased blood volume makes your heart work harder to move more blood through your blood vessels, increasing pressure in your arteries. If this becomes chronic, it can lead to heart disease, stroke, kidney disease and congestive heart failure.

Dietary guidelines recommend limiting sodium to less than 2,300 mg a day. The average American gets from 2,000 to 5,000 mg of sodium daily — much more than recommended and far more than our bodies need.

Dietary sources of sodium

The main sources of sodium in a typical diet include:

- **Processed and prepared foods.** This is where the vast majority of sodium comes from. Processed foods include prepared dinners such as pizza, pasta, meat and egg dishes, cold cuts and bacon, cheese, soups and fast foods. It's estimated that about 75% of your daily sodium intake comes from foods that have salt or sodium-containing compounds added during processing.
- **Natural sources.** Some unprocessed foods — including vegetables, milk, eggs, fresh meat and shellfish — naturally contain sodium. While these foods don't have an abundance of sodium, eating them does add to your overall sodium intake.
- **In the kitchen and at the table.** Many recipes call for salt, and many people also salt their food at the table. Condiments also may contain sodium. One tablespoon of soy sauce, for example, has about 900 mg of sodium.

So how can you tell which foods are high in sodium? Read food labels. The Nutrition Facts label found on most packaged and processed foods lists the amount of sodium in each serving. Other ways to limit sodium include eating more fresh foods, which are naturally low in sodium. You can also reduce the amount of salt in recipes and remove the saltshaker from the kitchen table. To add flavoring, use fresh or dried herbs, spices, onion or garlic instead.

FATS: THE GOOD AND THE BAD

Not all fats are created equal. There are different types of fat in the food you eat, and some are better for you than others.

- **Monounsaturated fat.** This type of fat is found in olive, canola and nut oils, as well as in nuts and avocados. Monounsaturated fat is considered a good fat. It helps lower blood cholesterol, and it's more resistant to oxidation. Oxidation is a process that promotes the buildup of fat and cholesterol deposits in the arteries. However, because all fat — even monounsaturated fat — is high in calories, you want to limit how much you eat.
- **Polyunsaturated fat.** Polyunsaturated fat is found in plant oils such as safflower, corn, sunflower, soy and cottonseed. It also includes omega-3 fatty acids found in fish. Polyunsaturated fat helps lower "bad" blood cholesterol, but it also lowers "good" blood cholesterol, and it seems susceptible to oxidation.
- **Saturated fat.** Saturated fat is an unhealthy fat that can raise your blood cholesterol and increase your risk of cardiovascular disease. It's found in meats and dairy products (including butter), as well as coconut, palm and other tropical oils.
- **Trans fat.** This type of fat was once found in stick margarine, shortening and processed products made from them, such as pastries, crackers, chips and other snack foods. The U.S. Food and Drug Administration (FDA) has banned food manufacturers from including trans fats — short for trans-fatty acids — in foods made or sold in the U.S. because of their harmful health effects. However, trace amounts may still be present. If "partially hydrogenated oil" is on the ingredients list, a small amount of trans fat may be lurking inside.

Keep in mind that your taste for salt is acquired. That means you can learn to enjoy less. Decrease your use of salt gradually, and your taste buds will adjust. After a few weeks of cutting back on salt, you probably won't miss it, and some foods may even taste too salty. Start by using no more than ¼ teaspoon of salt daily — at the table and in cooking. After a week or two, throw away the saltshaker. As you use less salt, your preference for it diminishes, allowing you to enjoy the taste of the food itself.

SMALL CHANGES ADD UP

We tend to get comfortable with our behaviors and habits. Even if they're not always healthy, they're familiar. They provide order and stability to our lives. That means most of us are reluctant to change the way we're used to doing things.

Although changes to your diet can be difficult, they're not impossible. And most people underestimate their ability to change. Changing behaviors in small ways can add up to a big difference in your health.

Here's a common dietary example: Many people have switched from drinking whole milk to skim milk. Maybe they tapered off gradually, or maybe they switched from one to the other in one bold leap. Either way, they made what they thought was an impossible change. Skim milk probably seemed watered down at first, but once used to skim, whole milk tasted too thick and rich. It's a small change, but if you drink two cups of milk a day, over the course of a year the simple step of switching from whole to skim can result in a loss of about 13 pounds!

Perhaps you've heard or read the statistic about the likelihood of keeping weight off permanently: 95% of individuals who lose weight regain it within five years. But this doesn't mean you're doomed to failure.

The National Weight Control Registry conducted a study involving 629 women and 155 men who had been overweight for years. The participants changed their eating and exercise habits, and they lost an average of 66 pounds each.

Some individuals eventually did gain some of the weight back, but they kept a minimum of 30 pounds off for at least five years. Most of them did it through a combination of exercise and a healthier diet — in other words, by changing their lifestyle. The participants also stated their weight loss improved their quality

UNPROCESSED VS. ULTRAPROCESSED FOODS

Most of the food that we eat today undergoes some sort of processing. That's not all bad, but it's important to understand the different types of processed foods. Some processing is necessary to make certain foods edible. But extensive processing can be harmful to your health. Food items that we eat today can generally be placed into one of four categories:

- **Unprocessed (natural) and minimally processed foods.** Unprocessed foods include things such as the edible parts of plants (seeds, fruits, leaves, stems, roots); the edible parts of animals (meat, eggs, milk); and things such as seafood, grains, nuts and mushrooms. Minimally processed foods are those that have been cooked or altered slightly in some way. Foods in this category are the ones that you want to eat the most of.
- **Processed culinary ingredients.** These are products extracted from nature and often used as seasonings. Examples are sea salt, molasses, honey, butter and pressed oils from olive, sunflower and other seeds. Some are combined, such as salted butter, and some have added vitamins, minerals or preservatives.
- **Processed foods.** Foods in this grouping include relatively simple products made by adding sugar, oil, salt or other processed culinary ingredients. The main purpose of processed foods is to increase the durability of unprocessed (natural) foods or to enhance their sensory qualities, such as taste. When you cook a homemade meal, for example, you are processing food. Processed foods also include those that have undergone various preservation methods, such as canning.
- **Ultraprocessed foods.** These foods undergo a higher level of processing. They're manufactured for convenience and taste. Ultraprocessed foods are generally high in sugar, oils, fats, salts and preservatives and contain little to no unprocessed (natural) foods. Some examples include soft drinks, frozen pizza, potato chips, prepackaged cookies, ice cream and prepackaged snacks. Ultraprocessed foods, in general, are very pro-inflammatory and can be damaging to your health. They are the foods that you want to avoid or keep to a minimum.

of life, including their mood, health and self-confidence. This group is living testimony that when you lose weight the right way — by making lifelong changes in your eating and exercise habits — you can be successful.

We mentioned in the previous chapter that our habits control at least half of what we do every day. More than 50% of the daily calories we consume are out of habit. A big part of improving your diet involves focusing on your habits.

And keep in mind that healthy eating is much more than what you eat or how much you eat. It's also about how you eat, whom you eat with, how fast or slow you eat, where you eat and what you're doing while you eat. These factors have tremendous influence on our eating habits.

Focusing on what you're eating — for instance, savoring food's textures and flavors and not being distracted by the television or your cellphone — allows you to eat at a slower pace, which promotes better portion control. There's usually about a 10-minute lag between when your stomach gets full and when your brain realizes it. The slower you eat and the more mindful you are of your surroundings and what you're eating, generally the less you eat.

The idea is that a meal should be an event — something that you look forward to and share with others when you can. Eating healthy doesn't have to be drudgery. It can, and should, be an enjoyable experience.

Holistic health to nurture your mind, body and spirit

CHAPTER | **16**

Building a solid wellness foundation means addressing all aspects of health — mind, body and spirit. As researchers continue to unravel the important role the mind plays in healing and fighting disease, it's becoming clear that good health stems not just from physical health but from overall well-being.

In previous chapters, you read how practices such as yoga and tai chi can encourage health and healing. And you learned the importance of social and emotional well-being — mind and spirit — to health and longevity.

Clearly, regular exercise and a healthy diet are vital to healthy aging. Researchers are also finding practices that nurture your mind and spirit may be equally beneficial. As part of your wellness plan, include activities that help reduce stress and anxiety, calm your mind, and promote relaxation and good sleep.

As evidence indicating the safety and effectiveness of many holistic practices grows, the practices are increasingly becoming integrated into conventional medical care.

MIND-BODY PRACTICES

Your mind and body are inextricably linked, meaning your thoughts and emotions can affect how your body functions. That's the premise behind mind-body interventions.

Traditional medicine has long concentrated on the biology of the body and brain. But that's changing. Over the past few decades, researchers and doctors have focused more attention on the effect the mind has on the body, particularly for diseases that appear to be brought on or exacerbated by stress, such as heart disease and asthma.

Practitioners of mind-body therapies believe that negative thoughts and feelings can produce bodily symptoms, including pain and muscle tension. To help relieve symptoms, they recommend relaxation techniques aimed at calming the mind as part of an overall wellness plan.

Keep in mind that these techniques often require practice. Be patient with yourself. As you learn the techniques, you'll become more aware of muscle tension and other physical sensations of stress. Once you know what the stress response feels like, you can make a conscious effort to practice a relaxation technique the moment you start to experience stress symptoms.

Progressive muscle relaxation

Progressive muscle relaxation is designed to reduce the tension in your muscles to help reduce stress, relieve headaches and clear your mind. It's easy to do and can be practiced just about anywhere.

You can practice muscle relaxation by itself or combine it with another mind-body approach, such as meditation. To perform progressive muscle relaxation, first find a quiet place where you can sit or lie down. Then, loosen any tight clothing and get comfortable. Beginning with your feet and working up through your body to your head and neck, tense each muscle group to the count of eight and then relax the muscles for up to 30 seconds. Do this a second time before moving to the next muscle group.

Yoga

You read about yoga earlier. It's an ancient practice that aims to induce physical, mental and spiritual well-being through a combination of postures (asanas), breathing techniques and meditation. It's increasingly popular among people seeking relaxation, a spiritual path or improvements in flexibility, coordination, balance, strength and endurance.

Research suggests that yoga may help reduce low-back pain, lessen stress, lower blood pressure, and help relieve anxiety, stress, depression and insomnia. It can also help improve overall physical fitness, strength and flexibility. At a minimum, yoga can relax you, and some forms may improve your physical conditioning.

With help from an experienced instructor, yoga is likely to help you and unlikely to be harmful. But yoga isn't easy. It requires discipline and concentration.

Meditation

Spending time each day meditating can help you relax, slow your breathing and heart rate and decrease muscle tension. Meditation can lessen your body's response to the chemicals it produces when you're stressed, such as adrenaline, which can raise your blood pressure and make your blood clot more easily — both of which raise your risk of heart disease.

Meditation helps you enter a deeply restful state in which you become very relaxed. The relaxation can help you manage pain and reduce stress and anxiety. During meditation, you sit still and make an effort to focus on a single thing, such as a particular word, phrase or sound. When your thoughts wander — as they inevitably do — you bring your focus back to where it was.

Various types of meditation are used to treat anxiety and stress. Meditation may help reduce high blood pressure and improve symptoms of fibromyalgia. For most conditions, though, additional research is needed to gain more conclusive results about the possible benefits of meditation. However, the practice is considered safe.

Guided imagery

Related to meditation, with this practice someone's voice, whether taped or live, directs you through a visualization exercise.

Once you reach a state of deep relaxation — most likely through meditation — you conjure up a visual image of whatever the person directing the exercise suggests. Perhaps it's a peaceful place, such as a colorful garden or a

ADDITIONAL WAYS TO COMBAT STRESS

There are many ways to manage stress. Experiment with the following strategies to see if they can help you deal with certain situations or circumstances that may cause you to feel pressured or anxious.

- **Make relaxation a daily habit.** Whether it be exercise, mind-body therapies, art, music or a hobby you enjoy, devote at least 30 minutes to these activities each day.
- **Simplify and organize your day.** If your busy lifestyle seems to be a source of stress, ask whether it's because you try to squeeze too many things into your day or because you aren't organized. If you're overextended, cut out some activities or delegate tasks to others.
- **Practice tolerance.** Try to become more tolerant of yourself and of situations over which you have little control. Remember that change is constant, and certain changes — losses, disappointments and events that you can't control — will continue to occur, like it or not.
- **Learn to manage anger.** Anger can significantly increase and prolong stress if you remain angry for an extended period. Anger can even trigger a heart attack. Identify your anger triggers and find release valves — ways to release the energy produced by your anger. Exercising, writing in a journal and listening to soothing music are a few ways to let go of anger.
- **Think positive.** In many cases, simply choosing to look at situations from a different perspective can reduce the stress in your life. Throughout the day, stop and evaluate what is causing you to think negatively about a certain situation and consider viewing it from a different perspective.
- **Seek professional help.** If these simple measures aren't helpful, don't be afraid to seek guidance from your health care provider, counselor, psychiatrist, psychologist or clergyperson. These people can provide you with additional and more personalized tools for recognizing and managing stress. Many people mistakenly believe that seeking outside help is a sign of weakness. To the contrary, it takes strength to realize that you need help and good judgment to seek it.

sandy beach, where you feel calm and safe.

Brain studies show that imagining something (visualizing) stimulates the same parts of your brain that are stimulated during the actual experience. If sitting by the ocean relaxes you, you may achieve the same level of relaxation by visualizing yourself there.

Deep breathing

This form of relaxation therapy focuses on deep, relaxed breathing as a way to relieve tension and stress. Deep breathing can be practiced most anywhere.

Begin by finding a comfortable position. It might be lying on a bed or couch or sitting in a chair. Then do the following:

- Inhale. With your mouth closed and your shoulders relaxed, inhale slowly and deeply through your nose to the count of six. Allow the air to fill your diaphragm — the muscle between your abdomen and chest — pushing your abdomen out.
- Pause for a second.
- Exhale. Slowly release air through your mouth as you count to six.
- Pause for a second.
- Repeat this breathing cycle several times.

Deep, or relaxed, breathing is a technique that helps you breathe more efficiently. It involves deep, even-paced breathing using your diaphragm to expand your lungs. The purpose of deep breathing is to slow your breathing, take in more oxygen and reduce the use of shoulder, neck and upper chest muscles while you breathe.

Practicing deep breathing produces several effects in your body, including the release of your body's natural painkillers — feel-good chemicals called endorphins — and increased blood flow to your major muscles. Deep breathing also makes it easier for your heart to do its work and helps your body and mind relax and regain strength and energy. It's generally a safe and easy mind-body approach.

Biofeedback

Biofeedback teaches you to control certain body functions, such as your heart rate. It's been shown to be effective in helping treat some medical conditions, as well as promote relaxation and relieve stress.

With biofeedback, you're connected to electrical sensors that allow you to receive information about your body.

This feedback helps you focus on making subtle changes, such as relaxing certain muscles, to achieve the results you want, which may be reducing tension, relieving pain or managing stress.

You can receive biofeedback training in physical therapy clinics, medical centers and hospitals, but biofeedback devices and programs are available for use at home, as well. Some of these are handheld portable devices, while others connect to your computer.

HANDS-ON PRACTICES

If you've ever had a massage, not to mention a hug from a friend or loved one, then you know how comforting human touch can be. Touch and manipulation of body tissues are at the core of several integrative treatments, often referred to as hands-on therapies.

Massage

Some people consider massage a luxury found in exotic spas and upscale health clubs. Not everyone is aware that massage — when combined with traditional medical treatments — is used to reduce stress and promote healing in people with certain health conditions.

Massage involves manipulation of your body's soft tissues — your skin, muscles and tendons. The type of manipulation — including its rhythm, intensity, rate and direction — varies with the type of massage, from the traditional kneading and rubbing in Swedish massage to the use of pressure at acupuncture points in shiatsu massage.

Almost everyone feels better after a massage. It's been shown to help relieve pain and soreness and reduce anxiety. Massage can also cause your body to release natural painkillers, and it may boost your immune system. If a massage causes discomfort, immediately inform the person who's performing it.

If you've been injured, consult your doctor before getting a massage. While generally safe, there are some instances in which a massage may not be recommended. These include having conditions such as burns or open wounds, deep vein thrombosis, unhealed fractures and severe osteoporosis.

Reflexology

The theory behind reflexology is that specific areas on the soles of your feet correspond to certain parts of your body — such as your head or neck or your internal organs. Reflexologists apply varying amounts of manual pressure to locations on the feet in an effort to influence a problem elsewhere in the body. The practice is sometimes combined with other hands-on therapies and may be offered by chiropractors or physical therapists.

There's little risk involved, and massaging the soles of your feet can feel good. While reflexology may promote relaxation, there's not much evidence to indicate it can treat disease.

Spinal manipulation

Spinal manipulation is based on the premise that health and disease are directly related to the functioning of the body's neuromusculoskeletal system, and with proper alignment of your bones, joints, muscles and associated nerves comes health and healing.

Spinal manipulation — also called spinal adjustment —is a technique in which practitioners use their hands or a device to apply a controlled thrust to a joint of your spine. Studies have found spinal manipulation to be an effective treatment for recent uncomplicated low-back pain. For this condition, short-term use of spinal manipulation has become an

accepted practice and is no longer considered alternative. But there's little evidence that long-term treatment is more effective than other therapies.

Studies also suggest spinal manipulation may be effective for headaches and other spine-related conditions, such as neck pain. There's no evidence, though, to support the belief that spinal manipulation can cure whatever ails you.

Spinal manipulation is generally considered to be safe, but it's not appropriate if you have osteoporosis or symptoms of nerve damage, such as numbness, tingling or loss of strength in a limb, hand or foot. Be cautious with the practice if you have a history of spinal surgery, vascular disease of the neck arteries or experience back pain accompanied by symptoms such as fever, chills, sweats or unintentional weight loss.

NATURAL ENERGY PRACTICES

Healing approaches that fit into this category are based on the idea that there's a natural energy that flows freely through your body or a field of energy that surrounds it. When this energy is disturbed or blocked, symptoms or disease may result. To treat the problem, energy flow needs to be restored.

WHAT ABOUT HERBS AND SUPPLEMENTS?

You can't help but notice them — the endless bottles of supplements that line the shelves of grocery and discount stores and drugstores, all promising to improve your health in various ways. The question is, do they actually work? Some may. Some don't. And for most, we simply don't know.

Millions of Americans take dietary supplements — pills, capsules and other forms — to promote health and healing. Because herbs are derived from plants, many people consider them natural and therefore assume they're safe. That's not necessarily so.

Vitamin, mineral and herbal supplements are all considered dietary supplements by the Food and Drug Administration. Unlike prescription and over-the-counter medications, which are tested rigorously to prove their benefits and identify their risks, most dietary supplements aren't. The fact is, you're far more likely to improve your diet and protect your health with good lifestyle habits than with dietary supplements.

Remember that their purpose is to supplement a healthy lifestyle, not substitute for one. Therefore, it's important to learn all that you can about any product you're using — or are considering using. If you want to take a vitamin or mineral supplement, here are some recommendations to keep in mind:

Read the label. The quality and strength of an herbal preparation can vary greatly by brand. When considering an herbal preparation, look for certifications or quality measures, such as those listed below. But be aware that these measures aren't always a guarantee against incorrect labeling.
- Current Good Manufacturing Practices from the FDA.
- International Organization for Standardization (ISO) 9000 or 9001.
- NSF certification, which comes from NSF International.
- A DNA barcoding program, which is used to identify herbal ingredients and to detect impure or unsafe ingredients in a dietary supplement.

Check where it's manufactured. Some supplements manufactured in other countries have been found to contain toxic ingredients — including lead, mercury and arsenic — and prescription drugs, such as prednisone.

Avoid supplements that provide megadoses. Most cases of nutrient toxicity stem from high-dose supplements. In general, choose a multivitamin-mineral supplement that provides about 100% Daily Value (DV) of all the vitamins and minerals. Taking significantly more than the recommended amount of some vitamins and minerals (megadoses) can be dangerous. The exception to the 100% DV recommendation is calcium. You may notice that calcium-containing supplements don't provide 100% DV. If they did, the tablets would be too large to swallow.

Beware of gimmicks. Don't give in to the temptation of added herbs, enzymes, amino acids or unusual "special" ingredients — they add nothing but cost.

Look for expiration dates. Supplements can lose potency over time, especially in hot and humid climates. If a supplement doesn't have an expiration date, don't buy it.

Follow directions. Don't exceed recommended dosages. In addition, some supplements can be harmful if taken for too long a time. Get advice from your doctor and other reputable resources.

Let your provider know what you're taking. Many people don't tell their health care providers they take dietary supplements because they think that their providers will disapprove or that it doesn't matter or because the providers don't ask. Tell your provider what you're taking, how often and how much. This is especially important if you have a health condition or are taking one or more medications. Some supplements can interfere with the action of prescription or over-the-counter drugs or have other harmful effects. If you're not sure if you need a supplement, ask your provider if you could benefit from an over-the-counter product.

Acupuncture

A component of Chinese traditional medicine, acupuncture has existed for at least 2,500 years. The philosophy behind it is that health depends on a vital energy called qi (pronounced CHEE) that circulates through your body along pathways called meridians. According to this ancient theory, if your qi is out of balance, you develop pain and disease. Inserting needles into specific points along the meridians unblocks the energy flow and restores your body's healthy balance.

When performed properly by trained practitioners, acupuncture has proved to be an effective therapy for:

- Pain, including chronic neck pain, chronic and acute low-back pain, knee pain, dental pain, osteoarthritis, labor pain, menstrual cramps and headaches.
- Nausea and vomiting in people who are receiving chemotherapy.

Although not completely proved, acupuncture may help relieve morning sickness in pregnancy. It's generally considered safe to have acupuncture when pregnant. However, let your acupuncture practitioner know you're pregnant, because certain acupuncture points that could stimulate labor and premature delivery need to be avoided.

Risks associated with acupuncture are low if you're working with a competent, certified acupuncture practitioner. The most common side effects include soreness, minor bleeding or bruising where the needles were inserted. However, acupuncture isn't suitable for everyone. You may be at risk of complications if you have a bleeding disorder. You should avoid the practice if you have a metal allergy. If you have a pacemaker, avoid acupuncture that includes mild electrical stimulation. The electrical pulses may interfere with the pacemaker's operation.

Acupressure is similar to acupuncture, but practitioners use their fingers instead of needles. The therapy involves pressing on specific acupuncture points in an attempt to help free the flow of natural energy.

Tai chi

An ancient Chinese tradition, tai chi is based on a series of slow, flowing movements that resemble a dance. It's designed to foster the free flow of energy that practitioners believe is necessary for good health. Today's practitioners use tai chi to gain emotional and physical balance, reduce stress and strengthen muscles and joints. Because it can help you feel both alert and tranquil, some people use it as a form of moving meditation.

Tai chi comprises hundreds of combinations of continuous movements that require concentration, balance and grace. When combined with deep, rhythmic breathing, these movements can increase circulation, relax your mind and body, and ease chronic pain. Practicing tai chi has been shown to improve balance, reducing the risk of falls.

Healing touch

Advocates of therapeutic touch subscribe to the notion that your body is its own form of energy, surrounded by a field of energy. Illness occurs when energy flow within and surrounding the body is blocked or congested.

During a healing touch session, practitioners typically move their hands over a person's body in the belief that they can get rid of the energy disturbance and transfer healing energy from their hands to the individual who's ill. The benefits of therapeutic touch aren't supported by solid research.

If you're new to mind and body practices, gather information, ask questions and feel comfortable with the answers you receive before taking part. Also keep in mind that some therapies may not be covered by insurance. Know what the therapy will cost you before you receive it.

CHARTING YOUR COURSE

As you move forward in your healthy aging journey, consider ways that holistic practices can play a role in your health. Think about the things that you do each day to enhance your well-being. Think of the things that you've learned from this book regarding physical activity, nutrition, stress management and social support. What do you do each day to support your wellness in these areas?

From eating the right foods and exercising regularly to meditating and getting a massage, every effort you make to improve your overall physical and mental health helps you and those around you. Healthy habits have a powerful ripple effect. Think about what you can do to integrate the best of complementary practices with the best of conventional medicine to achieve a lifetime of health and wellness.

Vaccinations and screening tests

Throughout this book, we mention that you should see your health care provider on a regular basis for basic preventive care. You may wonder, what does *regular* mean?

The answer depends on your age, your health and your family medical history. In general, if you're fairly healthy and you have no symptoms of disease, it's a good idea to have a physical 4 to 5 times in your 50s and then annually once you turn 60. More frequent visits may be advisable if you have certain health risks because of your personal or family health history.

Regular preventive exams are important because they help your health care provider assess your overall health and identify possible risk factors for disease that you may be able to modify. The payoff of these efforts can be a healthier and longer life.

Many conditions, such as diabetes, high blood pressure or some forms of cancer, don't present noticeable signs or symptoms in their early stages — but they may still be detectable with screening tests. Early detection is important. The sooner you know you have a disease, or may be at risk for it, the sooner you and your provider can take steps to manage and possibly even prevent the condition.

RECOMMENDED VACCINATIONS

One of the best ways to prevent most diseases and disorders is to make sure that you receive recommended vaccinations. Vaccines work by stimulating your body's natural defense mechanisms to resist infectious disease, destroying the disease-causing microbes before you become sick.

Most vaccinations are given in childhood. But there are some recommended

WHEN YOU SHOULDN'T 'WAIT AND SEE'

Oftentimes, when a particular sign or symptom develops, our natural response is to wait a day or two and see if it goes away. In many instances, such as if you develop a minor sore throat or you experience back pain after a day of lifting, this approach is OK. But certain signs and symptoms demand an immediate response. Seek emergency medical care if you experience any of the following:

- Uncontrolled bleeding.
- Difficulty breathing or shortness of breath.
- Severe chest or upper abdominal pain or pressure.
- Fainting, sudden dizziness or weakness.
- Weakening or numbness of an arm or leg.
- Sudden, marked change in vision.
- Confusion or changes in mental state.
- Any sudden or severe pain.
- Severe or persistent vomiting or diarrhea.
- Coughing or vomiting blood.
- Suicidal or homicidal feelings.

You may have other warning signs to be aware of given your personal medical history.

VACCINATIONS

Disease	What it is	
COVID-19	A viral disease that spreads easily from person to person.	
Hepatitis A	A viral infection of the liver transmitted primarily through contaminated food or water or close personal contact.	
Hepatitis B	A viral infection of the liver that's often transmitted through contaminated blood, sexual contact and prenatal exposure.	
Herpes zoster (shingles)	A viral infection that causes a painful rash. It's caused by the varicella-zoster virus — the same virus that causes chickenpox.	
Influenza (flu)	A respiratory disease that spreads from person to person when you inhale infected droplets from the air.	
Measles, mumps, rubella	Viral diseases that spread from person to person when you inhale infected droplets from the air.	
Meningococcal disease	A disease caused by bacteria that can cause meningitis, an inflammation of the membranes surrounding the brain and spinal cord.	
Pneumonia	An inflammation of the lungs, which can have various causes, such as bacteria or viruses.	
Respiratory syncytial virus (RSV)*	An infection of the lungs and respiratory tract spread from person to person primarily by inhaling infected droplets from the air.	
Tetanus and diphtheria or Tetanus, diphtheria and pertussis	Tetanus is a bacterial infection that develops in deep wounds. Diphtheria is a bacterial infection spread when you inhale infected droplets from the air. Whooping cough (pertussis) causes cold-like signs and symptoms and a persistent hacking cough.	

* Expected to be available Fall 2023

You're at increased risk if	Doses for adults
You're older, are immunocompromised or have certain medical conditions, including diabetes, cancer and chronic kidney, liver or lung disease.	One or two doses, depending on manufacturer. Additional primary doses or booster shots are recommended for certain individuals, including those at high risk.
You're traveling to a country without clean water or proper sewage, have chronic liver disease or a blood-clotting disorder, use illegal drugs or are male and gay.	Two or three doses depending on the vaccine. Avoid if you're hypersensitive to alum or 2-phenoxyethanol, a preservative.
Your occupation exposes you to blood and body fluids, you're on dialysis or have received blood products or you're sexually active with multiple partners.	Two, three or four doses depending on the vaccine or condition. Avoid if you're allergic to baker's yeast or if you've had a previous reaction.
You're older than age 50.	Two doses given 2 to 6 months apart.
You're age 50 or older, have a chronic disease or a weakened immune system, work in health care or have close contact with people who are at high risk of the disease.	One dose every year for all adults. Avoid if you're allergic to eggs or have had a previous reaction to a flu shot or history of Guillain-Barre syndrome within 6 weeks after previous dose of flu vaccine. A high-dose vaccine is available for adults ages 65 and older.
You were born after 1956 and don't have proof of previous vaccination or immunity.	One or two doses. Avoid if you received blood products in the past 11 months, have weakened immunity or are allergic to the antibiotic neomycin.
You have a compromised immune system or travel to certain foreign countries.	One or two doses can prevent a bacterial form of the illness.
You're age 65 or older, have a medical condition that increases your risk, such as chronic lung, liver or kidney disease or have a damaged or removed spleen.	One lifetime dose, but you may need a second dose if you're at higher risk or vaccination was before age 65.
You're older, have chronic heart or lung disease, have a weakened immune system or live in a long-term care facility.	One dose for adults age 60 and older based on discussions with a health care provider.
You suffered a deep or dirty cut or wound. You haven't received a previous pertussis vaccination — especially if you have close contact with an infant, for which pertussis is particularly risky.	Initial three-dose series (Td) with booster every 10 years. If your most recent booster was more than 5 years ago, get a booster after a wound. Initial three-dose series (Tdap) if you didn't finish the Td series as a child. Otherwise, one dose of Tdap when you're due for a Td booster, followed by a Td booster every 10 years.

specifically for adults or that may be recommended regularly throughout life. If you didn't receive a particular vaccination in childhood, it might still benefit you if given now.

When in doubt, follow your health care provider's advice on which vaccinations to receive and when to get them. He or she may recommend additional vaccinations depending on your occupation, hobbies or travel plans.

RECOMMENDED AND OPTIONAL SCREENINGS

Preventive screening exams are the best way to catch potential problems in their early stages — when the odds for successful treatment are greatest. In the pages that follow, you'll find information on exams or tests generally recommended for most adults and additional screening tests you may want to consider.

Remember, these are general guidelines. You and your health care provider should determine what tests are best for you and when to have them. For example, if you're older than age 50 or you're at risk of a particular disease, your provider may order additional tests or perform certain ones more frequently.

Blood cholesterol test

A blood cholesterol test is actually several blood tests (serum lipids). It measures total cholesterol in your blood as well as the levels of low-density lipoprotein (LDL, or "bad") cholesterol, high-density lipoprotein (HDL, or "good") cholesterol and other blood fats called triglycerides.

Triglycerides can raise your risk of heart disease. Levels that are borderline high (150 to 199 mg/dL) or high (200 mg/dL or more) may require treatment. Desirable levels are below 150 mg/dL.

What's the test for?

To measure the levels of cholesterol and triglycerides (lipids) in your blood. Undesirable lipid levels raise your risk of heart attack and stroke. Problems occur when your LDL cholesterol forms too many fatty deposits (plaques) on your artery walls or when your HDL cholesterol carries away too few.

When and how often should you have it?

Have a cholesterol evaluation at least every five years if the levels are within normal ranges. If the readings are abnormal, have your cholesterol checked more often. Cholesterol testing is especially important if you have a family history of high cholesterol or heart disease, are overweight, are physically inactive or have diabetes. These factors put you at increased disease risk.

What do the numbers mean?

The National Cholesterol Education Program has established guidelines to help determine which numbers are acceptable and which carry increased risk. However, desirable ranges vary,

BLOOD CHOLESTEROL NUMBERS

Total cholesterol level*	Total cholesterol category
Less than 200	Desirable
200 to 239	Borderline high
240 and above	High
LDL cholesterol level**	**LDL cholesterol category**
Less than 100	Optimal
100 to 129	Near optimal
130 to 159	Borderline high
160 to 189	High
190 and above	Very high
HDL* cholesterol level**	**HDL cholesterol category**
Less than 40 for men, less than 50 for women	Poor
40 to 59 for men, 50 to 59 for women	Better
60 and above	Best

*Numbers are expressed in milligrams of cholesterol per deciliter of blood (mg/dL).

**LDL means low-density lipoprotein.

***HDL means high-density lipoprotein.

Source: American College of Cardiology (2018), *Guideline on the Management of Blood Cholesterol.*

PREVENTIVE SCREENING EXAMS FOR WOMEN

Recommendations are based on average risk and normal results on prior testing.

Test	Ages 50 to 59	Ages 60 to 69	Ages 70 to 79	Age 80+
Blood cholesterol	At least every 5 years	At least every 5 years	At least every 5 years	At least every 5 years
Blood pressure	At least every 2 years	At least every 2 years	At least every 2 years	At least every 2 years
Bone density	Ask your provider	Screening at age 65	Ask your provider	Ask your provider
Clinical breast exam and mammogram	Every 2 years	Every 2 years	Every 2 years	Every 2 years
Colon cancer	Every 3-10 years (depends on test)	Every 3-10 years (depends on test)	Every 3-10 years (depends on test)	Ask your provider
Dental	Every 6 months to 1 year	Every 6 months to 1 year	Every 6 months to 1 year	Every 6 months to 1 year
Diabetes	Every 3 years	Every 3 years	Every 3 years	Every 3 years
Eye	Every 2-4 years; yearly if you wear glasses or contacts	Until age 65, every 2-4 years; beginning at age 65, every 1-2 years; yearly if you wear glasses or contacts	Every 1-2 years; yearly if you wear glasses or contacts	Every 1-2 years; yearly if you wear glasses or contacts
Pap test	Every 1-3 years, or longer depending on risk	Every 1-3 years through age 65; ask your provider	Ask your provider	Ask your provider

Other tests women should consider

Test	Ages 50 to 59	Ages 60 to 69	Ages 70 to 79	Age 80+
Hearing	Every 3 years	Every 3 years	Every 3 years	Every 3 years
Human papillomavirus (HPV)	Ask your provider	Ask your provider	Not necessary if you test negative up to age 65	Not necessary if you test negative up to age 65
Skin exam	Annually	Annually	Annually	Annually
Thyroid-stimulating hormone (TSH)	Ask your provider	Ask your provider	Ask your provider	Ask your provider
Transferrin saturation	Ask your provider	Ask your provider	Ask your provider	Ask your provider
Fall risk	Ask your provider	Ask your provider	Ask your provider	Ask your provider

PREVENTIVE SCREENING EXAMS FOR MEN

Recommendations are based on average risk and normal results on prior testing.

Test	Ages 50 to 59	Ages 60 to 69	Ages 70 to 79	Age 80+
Blood cholesterol	At least every 5 years	At least every 5 years	At least every 5 years	At least every 5 years
Blood pressure	At least every 2 years	At least every 2 years	At least every 2 years	At least every 2 years
Colon cancer	Every 3-10 years (depends on test)	Every 3-10 years (depends on test)	Every 3-10 years (depends on test)	Ask your provider
Dental	Every 6 months to 1 year	Every 6 months to 1 year	Every 6 months to 1 year	Every 6 months to 1 year
Diabetes	Every 3 years	Every 3 years	Every 3 years	Every 3 years
Eye	Every 2-4 years; yearly if you wear glasses or contacts	Until age 65, every 2-4 years; beginning at age 65, every 1-2 years; yearly if you wear glasses or contacts	Every 1-2 years; yearly if you wear glasses or contacts	Every 1-2 years; yearly if you wear glasses or contacts
Prostate-specific antigen (PSA) and digital rectal exam	Ask your provider	Ask your provider	Ask your provider	Ask your provider
Eye	Every 2-4 years; yearly if you wear glasses or contacts	Until age 65, every 2-4 years; beginning at age 65, every 1-2 years; yearly if you wear glasses or contacts	Every 1-2 years; yearly if you wear glasses or contacts	Every 1-2 years; yearly if you wear glasses or contacts

Other tests men should consider

Test	Ages 50 to 59	Ages 60 to 69	Ages 70 to 79	Age 80+
Hearing	Every 3 years	Every 3 years	Every 3 years	Every 3 years
Skin exam	Annually	Annually	Annually	Annually
Thyroid-stimulating hormone (TSH)	Ask your provider	Ask your provider	Ask your provider	Ask your provider
Transferrin saturation	Ask your provider	Ask your provider	Ask your provider	Ask your provider
Fall risk	Ask your provider	Ask your provider	Ask your provider	Ask your provider

depending on your individual health conditions, habits and family history. Talk with your doctor about what cholesterol levels are best for you and what you can do to maintain or achieve them.

Blood pressure measurement

This test — in which an inflatable cuff is placed around your arm — measures the peak pressure your heart generates when pumping blood out through your arteries (systolic pressure) and the amount of pressure in your arteries when your heart is at rest between beats (diastolic pressure).

What's the test for?

The test is used to detect high blood pressure. If you have increased blood pressure, the longer it goes undetected and untreated, the higher your risk of a number of diseases, including heart attack, stroke and kidney damage.

When and how often should you have it?

Have your blood pressure checked at least every two years. However, you'll probably have it checked every time you see a health care provider. If your blood

pressure is elevated, your provider may recommend more frequent testing. Testing is especially important if you have risk factors such as being Black, overweight or inactive, or you have a family history of the condition.

If your blood pressure is elevated, your provider may ask you to monitor it at home with a home blood pressure device. That's because blood pressure readings taken in a medical setting tend to be higher. Not all home devices are the same, so you should consult with your provider to ensure you purchase a device that's reliable and approved by the Food and Drug Administration.

What do the numbers mean?

An ideal or normal blood pressure for an adult of any age is a systolic pressure of less than 120 millimeters of mercury (mm Hg) and a diastolic pressure of less than 80 mm Hg.

Bone density measurement

A bone density test uses X-rays to measure how many grams of calcium and other minerals are packed into a segment of bone located in your lower back and hip region, wrist or heel.

What's the test for?

A bone density test is used to detect osteoporosis, a disease most commonly found in women that involves gradual loss of bone mass, making your bones more fragile and likely to fracture. Osteoporosis most often increases the risk of fractures of the hip, spine and wrist.

There are several different types of scans available. They include dual-energy X-ray absorptiometry (DXA) and computed tomography (CT).

When and how often should you have it?

Women should have a baseline exam after menopause, usually at age 65. However, if you have a family history of osteoporosis or other risk factors, earlier testing is a good idea.

In addition to older age, risk factors for osteoporosis include early menopause, frequent or extended use of steroid medications, smoking, low body weight and a history of fractures. Talk with your provider about a testing schedule that's right for you.

BLOOD PRESSURE NUMBERS

Top number (systolic)	Bottom number (diastolic)	Category
Lower than 120* and	lower than 80	Normal**
120 to 129 and	lower than 80	Elevated
130 to 139 or	80 to 89	Stage 1 hypertension
140 or higher or	90 or higher	Stage 2 hypertension
Higher than 180 and/or	higher than 120	Hypertensive crisis

*Numbers are expressed in millimeters of mercury (mm Hg).

**"Normal" means the preferred range in terms of cardiovascular risk.

Source: P. K. Whelton et al. (2017), *Guideline for the Prevention, Detection, Evaluation, and Management of High Blood Pressure in Adults.*

What do the numbers mean?

The T-score describes how much your bone density varies from what's considered normal. Normal is based on the typical bone mass of people in their 30s — the period in life when bone mass is at its peak. Peak bone mass varies from one person to another and is influenced by many factors, including heredity, sex and race. Men tend to have higher bone mass than do women, and white people and those of Asian descent generally have lower bone density than do people of Black and Latino ancestry.

- T-scores ranging from +1 or higher to -1 mean that your bone density is considered normal, and you're at low risk of bone fractures.
- T-scores ranging from -1 to -2½ indicate you have relatively low bone mass.
- T-scores of -2½ and lower indicate you have osteoporosis and are at greater risk of bone fractures.

Clinical breast exam and mammogram

These two tests are generally done in conjunction. A clinical breast exam is a physical check of a woman's breasts and armpits that's typically part of a routine physical examination. A mammogram is a screening test in which X-rays are taken of your breast tissue while your breasts are compressed between plates to spread the tissue apart.

What are the tests for?

The test is used to detect cancer and precancerous changes in your breasts. With a clinical breast exam, your doctor examines your breasts, looking for lumps, color changes, skin irregularities and changes in your nipples. Then your armpits are checked for swollen lymph nodes.

A mammogram can detect small breast lumps and calcifications — often the first indication of early-stage breast cancer — that are too small to be detected in a physical examination.

When and how often should you have them?

Before age 40, women should have a clinical breast exam at least every three years. For women age 40 and older, the exam is best done every year. Having regular breast exams is particularly important if you have a family history of breast cancer or other factors, including advanced age, that put you at increased risk of breast cancer.

There's some disagreement on the best screening schedule for mammograms. Proposed guidelines from the U.S. Preventive Services Task Force recommend that screening mammograms be done every two years beginning at age 40 for women at average risk of breast cancer. These guidelines differ slightly from those of the American Cancer Society (ACS). ACS guidelines call for yearly mammogram screening beginning at age 40 for women at average risk of breast cancer.

At Mayo Clinic, the current practice is to recommend an annual screening mammogram beginning at age 40, aligning with ACS recommendations. Screening mammography is not a perfect exam, but it's the best available tool to detect breast cancer early.

Talk with your health care provider about a schedule that's right for you. Regular mammograms are particularly important if you have a family history of breast cancer or have had prior abnormal breast biopsies.

If your breasts are sensitive, taking a pain reliever an hour or two before the test may help ease your discomfort. Avoid using underarm deodorant on the day of your mammogram as it affects the accuracy of the results.

Colon cancer screening

For this screening exam, a variety of tests may be used. You may have one or a combination of these colon cancer screening tests.

- **Colonoscopy.** During a colonoscopy exam, a long, flexible tube (colonoscope) is inserted into the rectum. A tiny video camera at the tip of the tube allows the doctor to detect changes or abnormalities inside the entire colon. Colonoscopy takes about 30 to 60 minutes, and screening is generally repeated every 10 years if no abnormalities are found and you don't have an increased risk of colon cancer.
- **Stool DNA test.** A stool DNA test uses a sample of your stool to look for DNA changes in cells that might indicate the presence of colon cancer or precancerous conditions. The stool DNA test also looks for signs of blood in your stool. For this test, you collect a stool sample at home and send it to a laboratory for testing. Stool DNA testing is typically repeated every three years.
- **Fecal occult blood test or fecal immunochemical test.** The fecal occult blood test (FOBT) and fecal immunochemical test (FIT) are lab tests used to check stool samples for hidden (occult) blood. The tests usually are repeated annually.

- **Virtual colonoscopy (CT colonography).** During a virtual colonoscopy, a CT scan produces cross-sectional images of the abdominal organs, allowing the doctor to detect changes or abnormalities in the colon and rectum. To help create clear images, a small tube (catheter) is placed inside your rectum to fill your colon with air or carbon dioxide. Virtual colonoscopy takes about 10 minutes and is generally repeated every five years.

What's the test for?

The test is used to detect cancer and precancerous growths (polyps) on the inside wall of the colon that could become cancerous. Some people are afraid of a colon cancer screening because they're embarrassed or worried the test will be uncomfortable. However, this screening could save your life by detecting and removing precancerous polyps, keeping cancer from developing.

When and how often should you have it?

If you're at average risk of developing colon cancer, have a screening test every 10 years beginning at age 45. The frequency of screening will depend on the type of test you have.

Talk with your health care provider about which screening approach and frequency are best for you, given your particular health issues. If you're at increased risk of developing colon cancer, your doctor may recommend that you start screening at an earlier age.

Dental checkup

Your dentist examines your teeth and checks your tongue, lips and mouth.

What's the test for?

A dental exam is done to detect tooth decay, problems such as tooth grinding and diseases such as periodontal disease. Your dentist also looks for lesions and other abnormalities in your mouth that could indicate cancer.

When and how often should you have it?

Have a dental checkup every six months to one year, or as your dentist recommends. Regular dental checkups are especially important if your drinking water doesn't contain fluoride or if you use tobacco or regularly drink alcoholic or high-sugar beverages or eat foods that are high in sugar.

Diabetes screening

Two blood tests are commonly used to screen for diabetes — a fasting blood sugar test and the A1C test.

A fasting blood sugar test measures the level of sugar (glucose) in your blood after you've fasted overnight or for at least eight hours.

An A1C test measures your average glucose level over the last two or three months by measuring what percentage of your hemoglobin — a protein in red blood cells that carries oxygen — is coated with sugar.

What's the test for?

Diabetes screening can detect high (elevated) glucose levels, which can damage your heart and circulatory system.

When and how often should you have it?

Have a baseline screening by age 45. If your results are normal, have your blood sugar rechecked every three years.

If you have a family history of diabetes or other risk factors such as obesity, your health care provider may recommend

DIABETES SCREENING NUMBERS

	Blood sugar level	A1C
Normal	Less than 100 milligrams per deciliter (mg/dL)	Below 5.7%
Prediabetes*	100 to 125 mg/dL	5.7% to 6.4%
Diabetes	126 mg/dL or higher on 2 separate tests	6.5% or higher on 2 separate tests

*Prediabetes means your blood sugar level is higher than normal and you're at increased risk of diabetes.

Source: American Diabetes Association, 2021

that you be tested at a younger age and more frequently. Screening is also recommended if you have signs and symptoms of diabetes, such as excessive thirst, frequent urination, unexplained weight loss, fatigue or slow-healing cuts or bruises.

What do the numbers mean?

A normal blood glucose level for an adult of any age is 70 to 100 milligrams of glucose per deciliter of blood (mg/dL). If your glucose level is greater than 125 mg/dL on two separate tests, you'll likely be diagnosed with diabetes.

For someone who doesn't have diabetes, a normal A1C level can range from 4.5% to 6%. An A1C level of 6.5% or higher on two separate tests indicates that you have diabetes.

Eye exam

During the exam, you read eye charts, look for specific visual images and may have your pupils dilated with eyedrops. An eye specialist also views the inside of your eye with an instrument called an ophthalmoscope and checks the pressure inside your eyeball with a painless procedure called tonometry.

What's the test for?

An eye exam allows your ophthalmologist or optometrist to check your vision and determine whether you may be at risk of developing vision problems.

When and how often should you have it?

If you wear glasses or contact lenses, have your eyes checked once a year. If you don't wear corrective lenses and have no risk factors for eye disease, have your eyes checked every 2 to 4 years until age 65. After age 65, it's best to have an exam every year or two.

Regular eye exams are especially important if you have diabetes, high blood pressure or a family history of glaucoma, cataracts or age-related macular degeneration.

Pap test

In this test, a health care provider inserts a plastic or metal speculum into the vagina to observe the cervix. Then, using a soft brush, the provider gently scrapes a few cells from the cervix, places the cells on a glass slide or in a bottle and sends the sample to a laboratory for analysis.

What's the test for?

The Pap test detects cancer and precancerous changes in the cervix. The test is usually done in conjunction with a pelvic exam. In women older than age 30, a Pap test may be combined with a test for human papillomavirus (HPV) — a common sexually transmitted infection that can cause cervical cancer. In some cases, the HPV test may be done instead of a Pap test.

When and how often should you have it?

Health care providers generally recommend Pap testing every three years for women ages 21 to 65. Women age 30 and older can consider Pap testing every five years if the procedure is combined with testing for HPV, or they might consider HPV testing instead of the Pap test.

Getting regular Pap tests is especially important if you smoke, have a sexually transmitted infection or multiple sex partners or have a history of cervical, vaginal or vulvar cancer. Your provider may recommend more frequent testing.

If you've had a total hysterectomy for a noncancerous condition, routine Pap tests aren't necessary. They're also not necessary if you're age 65 or older,

you've had normal test results over the past 10 years (including the last three tests) and you aren't at high risk of developing cervical cancer. When in doubt, ask your provider what's appropriate for you.

Prostate-specific antigen test and digital rectal exam

The prostate-specific antigen (PSA) test is a blood test that measures the amount of a specific protein secreted by the prostate gland. A digital rectal exam is a physical exam in which a health care provider feels the prostate gland for enlargement, tenderness, lumps or hard spots.

What are the tests for?

A digital rectal exam can detect prostate enlargement or prostate cancer. Don't be alarmed if your provider tells you that your prostate gland is enlarged. More than half of men older than age 50 have an enlarged prostate gland caused by a noncancerous condition called benign prostatic hyperplasia (BPH).

With the PSA test, increased PSA levels may indicate prostate cancer. However, other conditions can also elevate PSA.

When and how often should you have them?

Professional organizations vary in their recommendations about who should — and who shouldn't — get a PSA screening test. Organizations that recommend PSA screening encourage the test annually in men between the ages of 40 and 75 and in younger men with an increased risk of prostate cancer due to their race or family history. Talk with your provider about what's right for you.

What do the numbers mean?

The age-adjusted PSA scale in the box below shows the normal upper PSA limits, based on the PSA test used at Mayo Clinic. If your PSA level is above the normal upper limit for your age, talk with your provider about what your next

PROSTATE-SPECIFIC ANTIGEN (PSA) NUMBERS

Mayo Clinic urologists use this age-adjusted scale in determining if PSA results are within standard limits for your age. The results are based on the test used at Mayo Clinic. The upper limit of what's considered normal increases as you age.

Age	Upper limit
40 and under	2.0*
40-49	2.5
50-59	3.5
60-69	4.5
70-79	6.5
80 and above	7.2

*Numbers are expressed in nanograms per milliliter (ng/mL).

Source: Mayo Clinic.

step should be. Even if your PSA is normal but has recently increased substantially, further testing may be warranted.

Optional tests

The screening exams that follow are recommended for some individuals, depending on their health and personal risk factors. Talk with your provider to see if any of these tests may be appropriate for you.

Full-body skin examination

In this exam, a health care provider examines your skin from head to toe, looking for moles and spots that are irregularly shaped, have varied colors, are asymmetrical, are greater than the size of a pencil eraser, bleed or have changed since the previous visit.

The purpose of a skin examination is to check for signs of skin cancer or other skin changes that may put you at increased risk of skin cancer. You should have a full-body skin exam every three years in your 20s and 30s. Once you turn 40, have the exam every two years. Once you turn 50, have it every year.

Regular screening for skin cancer is especially important if you have many moles, fair skin, sun-damaged skin or a family history of skin cancer or if you had two or more blistering sunburns in childhood or adolescence. These factors put you at increased risk of developing skin cancer.

Hearing test

During a hearing test, a hearing specialist checks how well you recognize speech and sounds at various volumes and frequencies. The purpose of the test is to check for hearing loss, which becomes more common with increased age.

Have your hearing checked every 10 years until age 50. Starting at age 50, have it checked every three years. Hearing tests are especially important if you've been exposed to loud noises through your job or recreational activities, have had frequent ear infections or are older than age 60. These factors increase your risk of hearing loss.

Hepatitis screening

This is a simple blood test. The test is used to screen for chronic hepatitis B or

C. Hepatitis is an inflammation of the liver. People with chronic hepatitis B or C, caused by a viral infection, are at greater risk of liver disease and liver cancer.

Have a baseline test if you have one or more risk factors for hepatitis B or C. Risk factors include being exposed to human blood or body fluids, having multiple sex partners, receiving a blood transfusion before 1993 and living or traveling in an area where hepatitis B is common.

Human papillomavirus screening

This test is an additional screening option for cervical cancer that typically accompanies a Pap test. It's done to check for the presence of a high-risk strain of the human papillomavirus (HPV). Almost all cervical cancers are linked to infection by a high-risk strain of this virus. The HPV test involves the same method used to collect cervical cells during a Pap test; in fact, the test can be done at the same time.

If your Pap test indicates the presence of abnormal cells and you didn't have an accompanying HPV test, you should request one. Although there's no known cure for HPV infection, the cervical changes that result from it can be treated.

Thyroid-stimulating hormone test

This simple blood test measures the level of thyroid-stimulating hormone (TSH) in your blood, helping to determine whether your thyroid gland is functioning properly. TSH, made by the brain's pituitary gland, stimulates the thyroid gland to produce the hormone thyroxine. Sometimes, the thyroid produces too little thyroxine (possible hypothyroidism) or too much (possible hyperthyroidism).

Experts disagree about who can benefit from screening and at what age to begin. Talk with your provider about a screening schedule that's right for you. If you have high cholesterol, a family history of thyroid problems or symptoms of a thyroid condition, such as increased irritability or sluggishness, you may need more frequent testing than do others in the general population.

Transferrin saturation test

This simple blood test measures the amount of iron bound to an iron-carrying protein (transferrin) in your bloodstream. It can detect hemochromatosis, also called iron overload disease, a condition in which your body stores too much iron. Excessive iron can damage your organs and lead to diabetes, heart disease and liver disease. Hemochromatosis is an underrecognized but treatable hereditary disease.

Medical providers don't regularly test for hemochromatosis, but talk with your provider about testing if you have a family history of the disease or you have a condition that can be caused by hemochromatosis. They include joint disease, severe and continuing fatigue, heart disease, elevated liver enzymes, erectile dysfunction and diabetes. Some experts recommend a baseline test around age 30, with periodic repeat testing.

Fall risk assessment

For older adults, falls can be dangerous. Many people assume that falls are an inevitable part of aging, but they often can be prevented.

Health care providers use fall risk assessments to identify risk factors for falling and to make recommendations to help prevent them. Various medical organizations recommend that all adults age 65 and older have a fall risk assessment. For some people, a provider may repeat the assessment regularly.

Several tests and tools may be used to determine your fall risk, including an assessment of your balance, strength and pattern of walking (gait). If your provider feels that you may be at risk of falls, you may be asked to do the following:

- **30-second chair stand test.** For this assessment, you sit in a chair with your arms crossed to prevent you from using your arms for support. The individual performing the assessment keeps track of how many times you can stand up and sit down in a period of 30 seconds.
- **Timed Up & Go (TUG).** You begin by sitting in a chair with armrests. While being timed, you get up and walk 10 feet at your usual pace and return to the chair to sit down. The longer it takes to perform this exercise, the higher your fall risk.
- **Four-stage balance test.** You hold four different positions for 10 seconds each. The positions vary in difficulty, with the last one being standing on one foot.
- **Cognitive test.** You may undergo a brief cognitive assessment to check for any issues with thinking.

WORKING WITH YOUR PROVIDER

A key step in preventive health and overall management of your health is developing a good, ongoing relationship with a primary care provider who oversees all aspects of your medical care. Ideally, this person is someone who knows you and your family health history, as well as and the conditions under which you live and work that may affect your health.

IF YOU NEED SURGERY

News that you need to have surgery can prompt many questions and a lot of anxiety. Beyond details about your medical condition and treatment options, you'll probably want to know other things to feel comfortable with your care. In addition to helping to relieve your anxiety, the right surgeon and surgical center can reduce your risk of postoperative complications.

Here are five questions to ask your surgeon during your decision-making process:

1. **Are you board certified to perform this procedure?** Board certification is a credential that physicians earn in addition to state medical licensure. It means surgeons are qualified to perform a particular type of operation, such as cardio-vascular surgery.

2. **Will it help if I work on getting in shape before surgery?** Athletes know that the path to success is to be in the best of shape. The same holds true if you're heading into surgery. To help you prepare, your doctor may recommend prehabilitation. This is a period of time before surgery during which you work on improving your nutrition and building muscle. Even patients in wheelchairs have statistically better surgical outcomes if they undertake prehabilitation. Studies show that frailty is a risk factor for more complications and a longer stay in the hospital after surgery. If you're significantly overweight, losing weight could lower your risk for almost all major complications after surgery.

3. **Does it matter if I'm a smoker?** Smoking is a risk factor for many surgical complications, such as infections, slow healing, pneumonia and cardiovascular prob-

Optimal care generally results when you and your provider work as a team to identify the best course of care for you, a concept in health care called shared decision-making. The primary goals of a team approach are to get you and your provider on the same page regarding your health and how best to manage existing conditions, to avoid unnecessary or unsafe treatments, and to make sure that you're comfortable with the care that you receive.

lems. Even ending tobacco use just two weeks to a month before surgery can pay off. Sneaking a cigarette before surgery can mean a canceled operation. In some procedures, such as reconstructive cosmetic surgery with skin grafts, nicotine use raises the risk of a poor surgical outcome so much that you may be tested for nicotine the day of the operation; if the test is positive, the operation will be canceled until you're nicotine-free.

4. **What if I have sleep apnea?** Up to 1 in 5 older surgical patients has obstructive sleep apnea, and the breathing disorder has been associated with higher rates of post-surgery complications. If you have sleep apnea, make sure your surgeon knows that. If you're being treated with a continuous positive airway pressure (CPAP) machine, bring the machine with you for your hospital stay. And if you're at high risk of sleep apnea or worry about it, ask to be tested for sleep apnea before the operation.

5. **Is there anything we can do to shorten my hospital stay?** Steps to avoid complications will help reduce your hospital stay. Surgical site infections are a major preventable cause of prolonged hospitalization. A Mayo colorectal surgery study found that simply having patients shower with an antiseptic cleanser the day before and the day of surgery can help reduce infection risk. Ask your doctor if a minimally invasive procedure, with a shorter recovery time, is an option. Thanks to other improvements, such as less catheter use and new pain control methods that limit or eliminate opioid use, many patients are up and walking with assistance the night after surgery.

To help foster a good relationship with your provider, consider these steps:

- **Be on time for office appointments.** If you must cancel, try to do so at least 24 hours in advance. You may arrive for your appointment on time only to find that your provider is running late. Even so, you should be able to see your provider within a reasonable amount of time. However, realize that this person may occasionally be called away to address medical emergencies.

- **Be prepared for your appointments.** Before each visit, jot down a couple of main problems that are of concern to you. Be ready to bring up relevant changes in your personal or family health history.

- **Answer all your doctor's questions truthfully and completely.** This helps your provider better monitor your health, assess any health risks you may have and make a proper diagnosis, if one is needed. Even if the subject is sensitive, such as smoking, alcohol or drug use or sex, be truthful. To help you, your provider needs an accurate picture of what's going on in your life.

- **Make sure you understand what's been said.** If you don't understand something, ask your provider to clarify it for you until you do understand. You should know what your provider is recommending and why. If you think you may not remember, write it down.

- **Follow treatment recommendations.** If you're prescribed a medication or another form of treatment, do what is being recommended. Be patient; sometimes a treatment takes time to take effect. However, if you experience any adverse effects or your symptoms get worse, contact your provider.

MANAGING YOUR MEDICATIONS

If you're fortunate, you don't have to take any medications. But the fact is, as you get older, the chances that you'll need to take a medication increase. Medications serve a vital role in maintaining good health, and taking a drug doesn't mean that your health is poor. But almost anything with the power to heal also carries the power to harm when used incorrectly.

If you take medication regularly, remember these important tips:

- **Keep your provider up to date.** Be sure your health care provider knows about all the medications you're taking, including over-the-counter medicines, vitamins and supplements. Before your appointments, list the medications you've been prescribed by all your doctors and the vitamins and supplements you take or bring the bottles with you (including over-the-counter and nonprescription drugs). Having this information allows your doctor to make sure that products aren't adversely interacting with each other.

- **Know what you're taking and why.** For each medication you take, you should know what it is, why you're taking it, how to take it and for how long. It may be helpful to create a medication log and carry it with you.
- **Beware of polypharmacy.** As you age, your body may react to medication differently than when you were younger. That can be a problem, particularly if you have multiple prescriptions. Taking five or more drugs is called polypharmacy and it can lead to what's known as a prescribing cascade. That's when a doctor mistakes a medication side effect for a new condition and prescribes something else to treat it. Studies show the more medications you take, the more likely you are to have a side effect.
- **Don't pharmacy-shop.** If possible, use one pharmacy to fill all your prescriptions. This will help your pharmacist detect whether there are duplications or potential adverse interactions in your medications. If any instructions on a medication label are unclear, ask your pharmacist to clarify. If your prescription looks different from what you expected, inquire about it.

- **Take your medication as directed.** Don't stop taking it just because you're feeling better, unless your doctor instructs you to do so.
- **Avoid interactions.** Don't take medications with alcohol, hot drinks or vitamin or mineral supplements. These combinations may cause adverse drug interactions. Also, don't stir drugs into food unless advised to do so.
- **Keep your medications in a safe location.** Don't store your medications in the bathroom, near the kitchen sink, on a windowsill or in your car. Moisture, heat and direct light can change a medication's strength. Better storage options are a high kitchen cabinet or bedroom dresser drawer, out of the reach of children and pets. Also, keep your medications in their original containers.

Even nonprescription medications can cause side effects and be dangerous if misused. Follow the same safety precautions for over-the-counter products, including supplements, as you do for prescription medications. For more information on safe use of supplements, see pages 268-269.

Planning ahead for what comes next

18

Retirement is sometimes referred to as the third phase of life. Traditionally, it's the time when a person's working years end and they set sail — literally or figuratively — for new horizons. Many people spend decades imagining what they'll be doing for the rest of their lives beyond their careers. The reality is that how well you'll do in your later years is often tied to how well you've planned for them.

If you haven't done much planning and you retire with limited income and health insurance that doesn't cover your medical needs, your retirement years may be stressful.

With good planning, you can avoid many of the hassles that can create hardship in peoples' later years. You don't have to retire rich, but you want to make sure

you have your finances, health insurance and living arrangements in order so you can enjoy this phase of your life. Taking care of key paperwork, such as advance directives, is another important step.

Retirement simply isn't what it was for our parents and grandparents. Many Americans who retire today in their mid-60s still have one-quarter to one-third of their lives to live after retirement. In contrast, when Social Security was launched in 1935, life expectancy was about 63, so most people just lived a few years after retirement.

Retirement today is different. And with so many years to spend in this next phase of your life, you need activities to fill your day and money to live on.

That's why the prospect of retirement is both exciting and scary for many people: Exciting because of the many opportunities it presents — pursuit of new interests and hobbies, travel and adventure, more time to spend with family and friends — and scary because of the financial issues involved and the retooling of your lifestyle that retirement may pose.

No matter your age, it's never too early to start planning for retirement. In fact, the earlier you start the better. Making your dreams a reality and dealing with other issues associated with your later years takes some very down-to-earth work, which generally is best done in advance.

This chapter focuses on things that you should be thinking about before you retire to help make the transition to retirement a smooth one.

ARE YOU READY TO RETIRE?

There isn't a one-size-fits-all best age at which to retire. Many factors — positive and negative — can affect the timing of this major life decision. Concerns about job-related stress, health issues, financial risks, professional identity and social connections can color your perception about when it feels right to step away from work.

In Chapter 13, you learned about strategies to help you cope with major life transitions such as retirement. That chapter includes information on how to reduce anxiety, build a support network and find your purpose in this next phase of life — important issues as you consider retirement.

For most individuals, however, one of the key factors in determining when they'll retire is whether they can afford to do so. Financial security is perhaps the biggest concern, and source of stress, in planning for retirement.

FINANCIAL PLANNING AND YOUR HEALTH

It's well-known that money doesn't buy happiness before or after retirement. But not having enough money can be a major source of stress, and the stress of not having adequate financial resources can affect your health.

Research indicates that people with sound finances generally cope better with illness than do people who don't have the funds they need. Likely reasons are that they're not burdened by the cost of their medical care, and they experience less stress and anxiety in managing their illnesses. Along with healthy habits, such as diet, exercise and social ties, having adequate financial resources is a component of well-being. Again, you don't need to be wealthy, but you want to have a feeling of financial security.

Retirement calculators — perhaps from your place of employment or from organizations such as AARP — can help you determine whether you have the financial wherewithal to retire. By answering a few questions about your household, salary and retirement savings, you can get a personalized assessment of how much money you'll need in retirement and if you have enough money saved up. You might also consider talking to a financial advisor.

Government statistics indicate that the average American retires at age 67. With longevity increasing, that means it's wise to plan for savings sufficient to last 30 years, so that you don't outlive your income. When you reach 10 years from your anticipated retirement date, take stock of where you stand financially in case you need to make adjustments to your savings plan.

In plotting a timeline for your retirement, take note of these age-specific milestones:

- You can start making catch-up contributions to your 401(k) or 403b and other defined contribution retirement accounts at age 50.
- At age 59½, you'll no longer be penalized for early withdrawals from retirement accounts.
- You can start taking Social Security at age 62, but your monthly benefit will be higher if you wait.
- Medicare eligibility begins at age 65.
- You have to start taking minimum withdrawals from most retirement accounts at age 72.

It's impossible to predict exactly how your retirement will go, but a realistic plan can increase your odds of achieving your goals and dreams. People who plan ahead generally have more resources when they're ready to retire. Once you establish your basic goals — including your retirement age, the lifestyle you want and the income you'll need — then you can plot out how to achieve them.

HOUSING

Another important decision that often comes with retirement is where you want to live in your later years. Some retirees sell their house and move to a warmer climate or a retirement community. Others prefer to stay in their home or to stay in the area but downsize. The decision about where to live and whether to move can be a complex one that involves economics, lifestyle preferences and available resources.

Your current home is the place you likely feel the most comfortable, safe and secure. Maybe you've already paid off your mortgage, so except for taxes and maintenance, your housing costs are limited. Perhaps you've rented an apartment for years, and it's home and you really can't see moving.

Take an objective look at your current residence to be sure it makes sense for the long term. Most homes in the United States are designed for able-bodied occupants and may not accommodate the needs of someone who needs to use a device such as a wheelchair to get around.

Consider, for example, whether the stairs of your two-story home might eventually present a problem. Is the only bathroom on the second floor? Is the laundry in the basement? Is upkeep of a big backyard likely to become a burden? Major repairs may also become common as plumbing and heating systems age and wear out.

If you want to stay in your home, you may need to make some modifications to make it more convenient and accessible. Do you have the money to do that?

A cold, hard look at your home might convince you that it's time to move while you're still in good physical health. Maybe a single-story ranch makes more sense, or maybe all you really need is a two-bedroom home. Downscaling could ease your expenses. Standard apartments, condominiums and town houses can provide the living space you need without the worries of exterior upkeep; nearby neighbors can offer social and safety advantages as well.

Retirement communities

Retirement communities are popular and provide a variety of options for independence. Often, they're multi-unit complexes of condos, town houses or apartments. One of the major benefits of a retirement community is the reduced hassle of home ownership. Such a facility draws like-minded older adults together and delivers the community services that residents most want and need.

Continuing-care retirement communities go even further. These facilities offer multiple services on an a la carte basis so that as residents' needs change, they can receive additional services within the same setting. A retirement community may provide the independent living setting that you want now and the assisted living setting you may need in the future.

Shared living

Despite the freedom living alone offers, it isn't for everyone. There are some real

---

KEY RETIREMENT QUESTIONS

Making a checklist can be helpful as a jumping-off point for planning your retirement, plus it's a tool that you can revisit as the actual date approaches. You might visit with a financial planner to help you develop a retirement plan that meets your goals and fits within your expected income.

Here are some questions to consider:

- What are your personal and financial objectives for retirement? Do you want to travel, and if so, how much? Do you want to build a home or move to a different area? You should have some idea of what your dreams will cost to make sure that you have enough money saved up.
- What will your estimated monthly and annual *necessary* expenses be during retirement? How much will the *nonessential* things you'd like cost?
- When will you take Social Security?
- How will you pay for routine health care?
- If you need home health care or care in a skilled nursing facility, how will you pay for it?
- How will you provide for any dependents that outlive you?
- Do you have a will and an advanced care directive?

advantages, both for your emotional well-being and your physical safety, to sharing your own residence or moving in with another person or group of like-minded individuals.

Sharing your home or joining someone else in their home can be a joy, a disaster or something in between. Consider any arrangement on a trial basis to start, and have open discussions beforehand about issues such as rent, cooking, cleaning, maintenance and personal space.

Moving in with younger family members used to be the way most older adults transitioned out of their homes. But with today's far-flung families, that's not

RESOURCES FOR INDEPENDENT LIVING

Part of living independently means recognizing limitations that present themselves and seeking help in managing them. Below is a list of services to help you live independently and stay productive for many years to come.

- **Home health care.** Some health care services can be provided at home by trained professionals, such as home health nurses.
- **Household maintenance.** While staying in your house may be appealing, certain tasks may become difficult with time. Look for people or resources in your community that can help with housekeeping, shopping or handyman services.
- **Personal care.** This involves help with daily living, such as dressing, bathing or meal preparation. You might hire a personal care aide or home health aide.
- **Social interaction.** Feelings of isolation may crop up from time to time. Your local senior and community centers are excellent resources for recreational and educational activities that can keep you socially involved. Some may have day care options for adults with greater health and social needs.

A great place to start searching for resources in your area is the Eldercare Locator provided by the U.S. Administration on Aging. See page 320 for additional information.

always an option. If you want to live with your children or they're urging you to move in with them, have frank discussions about each other's expectations. Consider everything from partner and spouse relationships and finances to living space allocations and childcare before you start packing.

Assisted living

Assisted living can be a great option if you need some assistance with bathing, dressing, meal preparation and housekeeping. It is a valid alternative to hiring private help in your own home. Assisted living centers usually offer a menu of options, allowing you to tailor the services and costs to your specific needs.

Many assisted living arrangements charge a monthly rental fee for an apartment with utilities, meals, housekeeping, laundry and an emergency call system provided. Additional services generally include extra fees.

Fully supported living

Most people prefer to live in their own homes. But health conditions may dictate the need for fully supported care, such as that offered by a skilled

nursing facility. U.S. Census Bureau and other national figures indicate that only about 15% of Americans age 85 and older live in a skilled nursing facility. The average skilled nursing facility resident has several chronic illnesses that require medical attention.

When independent living, assisted living or care by family members isn't feasible or threatens to destroy the fabric of a family, you may have to consider a skilled nursing facility. In terms of your independence, you will undoubtedly experience some feelings of compromise should you eventually need to move to a fully supported care facility. But you still have the power to choose how you think about those challenges and how they shape your outlook on life.

MEDICARE

As you enter your second 50 years — the time in your life when you're most likely to need medical care — it's essential that you have appropriate health insurance. Having good health insurance is more than just a smart financial move. Good insurance can also affect your health. How so? You're more likely to see a doctor for preventive care and when problems arise if you know that your insurance will cover the cost. This results in earlier diagnosis and treatment of illness, which is typically when the chances of a cure are greatest.

Good health insurance also reduces stress. Instead of worrying how you'll pay your latest bill, you can concentrate on other more enjoyable — and less stressful — matters. And it's reassuring to know that if a health problem does occur, you're covered.

Many people don't retire until age 65 because that's the year they become eligible for Medicare. Medicare is the federal health insurance program for U.S. citizens age 65 and older. It also provides health insurance to individuals under age 65 who have a disability that prevents them from being employed. You're eligible for Medicare no matter how much money you have.

Medicare basically has two main components, Part A and Part B. Because Medicare won't cover all of your health care expenses, there are a number of options to supplement your basic Medicare insurance.

Medicare Part A

If you're already receiving Social Security benefits, you're automatically enrolled in Medicare Part A. Even if your Social Security benefits don't begin until a later age or you don't plan on retiring until later, you're still eligible for Medicare at age 65. Part A pays for most of these services:

- Hospital stays in a semiprivate room, including mental health care.
- Post-hospitalization skilled nursing care, including rehabilitative services, for a limited time.
- Home health care visits from a nurse or therapist and durable medical equipment such as a wheelchair or hospital bed.
- Hospice care, including drugs for pain relief and symptom control.

Medicare Part B

Medicare Part B pays for some or most of these services:

- Visits to your health care providers. This includes a one-time "Welcome to Medicare" preventive visit within the first year of obtaining Part B, and a yearly wellness visit to assess your health and risk factors once you've had Part B for more than 12 months.
- Outpatient hospital care, including outpatient physical or speech therapy.
- COVID-19, flu and pneumococcal vaccinations and hepatitis B vaccinations for people at high risk.

- Second opinions for nonemergency surgery.
- Laboratory services.
- Some medical equipment and supplies.

- Preventive screenings, including mammograms and colonoscopies.
- Adult care, mental health treatment and some counseling.

FINDING OUT MORE ABOUT MEDICARE

Navigating the ins and outs of Medicare and all its plans can be an overwhelming task, but there are a number of resources to help you:

Medicare's website. Medicare has an interactive online tool called the Medicare Plan Finder, which lists Medigap, Medicare Advantage and other supplemental policies in your ZIP code. The organization also has a number of helpful publications. You can get free copies by visiting Medicare's website, www.medicare.gov. An additional portal on the Medicare site provides free access to personalized information about your current Medicare benefits and services.

State health insurance department. Every state has a program — often called the state health insurance assistance program (SHIP) — to help people sort out Medicare issues, Medigap policies and managed care plans. SHIP staff not only can assist you with information regarding Medicare but also may often be able to help you sift through various policies, assessing the pros and cons of each. You can find your local SHIP at www.shiphelp.org/.

Insurance agent. An insurance agent can help you find a supplemental health insurance policy, but most agents recommend only certain companies. For a broad selection, talk to more than one insurance agent.

Friends and family. Ask around. Your friends and extended family members may be able to give you valuable firsthand reports on how well different Medicare plans fit their needs.

- Home health care.
- Alzheimer's-related therapy.
- Weight-loss therapy.
- Tobacco cessation counseling.

Part B does not cover:
- Treatment that isn't medically necessary, such as cosmetic surgery or alternative therapies.
- Other vaccinations.
- Most medications, with the exception of some administered by a medical professional, such as some immunosuppressant, anticancer and dialysis drugs.
- Hearing and routine eye exams.
- General dental work or dentures.
- Acupuncture.

Getting Medicare coverage

It's important to do your homework, because Medicare offers several types of health plans, with varying amounts of coverage and costs. Keep in mind that no matter which you pick, you're still in the Medicare program.

Original Medicare

This is the traditional basic plan you're automatically enrolled in unless you choose another privately funded option.

It pays Medicare's share of your costs under Parts A and B. You pay the balance. You receive all of the services Medicare covers, but no extra benefits.

Medigap policies

Medicare isn't designed to cover all of your medical expenses, so you may want to purchase a supplemental insurance policy. Medigap policies pay for gaps in coverage — things that Original Medicare doesn't pay for. There are many different types of Medigap policies, and their availability varies, depending on your insurance company and state laws.

Some policies help pay limited amounts for prescription drugs, but policies sold after Jan. 1, 2006, aren't allowed to include prescription drug coverage. Instead, you're eligible to participate in the Medicare Prescription Drug Plan — otherwise known as Medicare Part D for drug coverage.

You only need one Medigap policy to supplement your Original Medicare plan. In fact, it's illegal for an insurance company to sell you a policy that duplicates coverage you already have. Remember that your Medigap policy applies only to you. You and your spouse must purchase separate Medigap policies.

Medicare Advantage (Medicare Part C)

This is also designed to cover gaps in Original Medicare. But with this choice, you receive your health care entirely through a managed care plan. Some managed care plans charge no premium at all. You don't need a separate Medigap policy if you join a Medicare managed care plan, because the managed care plan agrees to cover some of the same services as Medigap plans.

Private fee-for-service (PFFS) plans

This is private insurance that accepts Medicare beneficiaries. Private fee-for-service plans offer more flexibility than managed care plans in that you're not restricted to particular networks of health care providers — you can see any doctor or go to any hospital in the country that accepts the plan's payment terms. However, in return for this flexibility, you typically pay higher premiums and out-of-pocket expenses.

Special needs plans (SNP)

These focus on specific groups of people, such as individuals in long-term care facilities or people with a particular chronic disease such as cancer or dementia. The plans seek to provide more targeted health care to meet the special needs of a covered group in a more efficient and effective manner. To find out if any specialty plans are available in your area, call Medicare or log on to its website (see page 321).

Prescription drug plans (Medicare Part D)

These offer coverage for the cost of some prescription drugs through private companies. These plans are voluntary, and to enroll, you must have Medicare Part A or Part B. The drug coverage may come as part of a Medicare Advantage (Part C) plan or as a stand-alone plan that works with Original Medicare.

Other options, including prescription drug plans with smaller premiums and lower deductibles, are also available.

Making a decision

To determine which plan is the best for you, keep the following points in mind:

Coverage away from home

If you travel often or you live in another part of the country for part of the year, make sure that your plan covers you while you're away from home. Managed care plans offer only limited coverage while you're away from home.

In addition, Medicare doesn't cover care received in a foreign country, although some private health insurance plans may provide this benefit. If you're taking a trip outside the country, you may wish to purchase a temporary, one-time health insurance policy that will cover you while you're away. These are often available through a travel agent.

Specialists when you want them

Medigap and fee-for-service plans let you see any specialist whenever you want to. Most managed care plans require you to see specialists who are part of the plan's network. Often you must get a referral first. Make sure the specialists that you want to see are part of your plan's network. If they aren't, you'll pay much more out-of-pocket when you see them.

Limited budget

Medicaid is a government program that helps people with low incomes pay medical bills. To qualify for Medicaid, you and your spouse must have a low income and few assets. If you're eligible for Medicaid, it acts like a Medigap policy. The lower your income and assets are, the more Medicaid helps pay for your Medicare out-of-pocket expenses. Medicaid also pays for skilled nursing facilities and other long-term care.

Each state has different Medicaid rules. To find out if you qualify in your state, call your state's department of social or human services.

Employer-based coverage

Not everyone retires at age 65, so you may still be receiving health insurance coverage from your employer when you become eligible for Medicare. Usually, employers require that you sign up for basic Medicare when you become eligible but offer their group health insurance benefits in conjunction with Medicare.

Some companies offer health insurance benefits as part of a retirement package. Even if you're eligible for work-related health insurance, it may be worthwhile to compare plans offered through your current or former employer with Medicare plans to see which offers the best value.

LONG-TERM CARE INSURANCE

Long-term care insurance covers services that you may need, including skilled nursing facility care, if you're unable to care for yourself because of a prolonged illness or disability. This insurance can provide some financial protection if you're diagnosed with a chronic illness, disability or mental impairment, such as Alzheimer's disease, and need long-term care. Long-term care

TRAVEL MEDICINE

With more flexible time on their hands, many retired individuals enjoy traveling. Travel can sometimes require significant preparation, even for the most experienced traveler. Beyond the usual challenges of booking, you may need to plan for your medication and medical equipment while away from home. It's also important to know where and how you can get medical care if you become ill or are injured.

The Centers for Disease Control and Prevention (CDC) recommends that if you travel internationally, make an appointment with your health care provider to get destination-specific vaccines, medicines and information at least a month before you leave. Let your provider know where you're going and what type of activities you're planning. The CDC also recommends that you purchase travel insurance.

Be sure to pack all the medications you need for your trip in a carry-on bag. Take with you a list of your prescriptions and over-the-counter supplements and their dosages and your doctor's contact information in case of an emergency.

If you'll be sitting for a long time on a plane or in a train or car, consider wearing compression stockings to help prevent blood clots (deep vein thrombosis). It's also a good idea to walk or stretch your legs if possible. Masking if you're on a plane or train is a good idea to prevent infection, as well as washing your hands before taking off your mask to eat.

generally covers a wide variety of services, from the cost of home health care to monthly skilled nursing facility payments.

Long-term care is often expensive and generally isn't covered by Medicare. When thinking about long-term care insurance, it's important to consider all the pros and cons.

Do you need it?

People buy long-term care insurance for the following reasons:
- To pay for significant care, thus protecting assets they plan to leave to their heirs.
- To prevent their family members from having to take care of them or paying their medical bills.
- To avoid becoming dependent on the government for their care.

People also purchase long-term care insurance for peace of mind, knowing the cost of their care will be covered if needed.

Most individuals, however, never end up staying in skilled nursing facilities; of those who do, the majority are there for only a short time. This is not to say that long-term care insurance can't be useful.

Such insurance may help with other types of care, especially home health care or assisted living. But long-term care insurance isn't the best choice for everyone, and knowing the facts will help you in your purchasing decisions.

Who should buy it and when?

A long-term care insurance policy is most appropriate for people whose income is in the middle-class range and who have a limited amount of assets they want to protect. If you are considering purchasing long-term care, keep these points in mind:
- As a general rule, you shouldn't spend more than 5% to 7% of your annual income to pay for premiums.
- Don't purchase a policy if paying the premium forces you to change your lifestyle or if you can't afford premium increases of 20% to 30% during the policy's lifetime.

In general, the younger you are when you purchase a long-term care insurance policy, the lower your premiums will be. But if you buy it too young, you may pay many years of unnecessary premiums.

Long-term care insurance can be complicated. If you have questions about whether long-term care insurance is right for you, you may want to consult a financial adviser. He or she can help you sort through the pros and cons on the basis of your finances and help you understand the fine print.

ADVANCE DIRECTIVES

With the advent of newer medications, surgical techniques and life-sustaining technologies, medicine has become increasingly capable of prolonging life. Sometimes, death due to natural heart, lung or other organ failure can be postponed with these measures.

One of the most important things that you can do with your doctor and your family is to have a frank discussion about how you wish to be treated when you don't have the capacity to make decisions for yourself, such as when you're unconscious or too sick to communicate. In circumstances such as these, an advance directive can guide your family and caregivers in carrying out your preferences regarding your care.

An advance directive is a legal document that spells out the types of medical treatments and life-sustaining measures you do or do not want. It may also specify whom you've appointed to make medical decisions on your behalf. In some states, this type of document may be known by a different name, such as a health care directive or health care declaration.

If you're older than age 18 and admitted to a hospital, skilled nursing facility, hospice or home health care agency that receives Medicare funds, the institution is required by federal law to ask whether you have an advance directive. That information is documented in your record. In the absence of an advance directive, a doctor will rely on your next of kin for guidance.

A medical institution that receives Medicare funds must also provide you written information about your right to accept or reject medical treatment. Whether or not you have an advance directive, federal law requires that medical institutions provide all individuals the same treatment options.

Types

The most common types of advance directives are a durable power of attorney for health care and a living will. A combination of the two provides your maximum personal participation in the face of medical situations that require difficult decisions to be made.

Durable power of attorney for health care

This document indicates whom you trust to make health-related decisions for you, should you become unable or unwilling to do so. The individuals you name have legal authority to act on your behalf to help ensure that your wishes about your care aren't misinterpreted or ignored.

Don't confuse a durable power of attorney for health care with a financial power of attorney. A financial power of attorney is a document in which you authorize one or more persons to manage your money and property if you aren't able to do so.

Living will

This document specifies which medical treatments you want or don't want at the end of your life. Because no one can anticipate all of the possible circumstances surrounding your death, it's hard to be specific in living wills.

For example, you may state that you don't want heroic procedures to extend your life when death is imminent, but your doctor still has to make certain distinctions as necessary: Is the use of a respirator a heroic measure? What about a blood transfusion?

Preparing and changing your directives

You may want to enlist an attorney to help you prepare an advance directive, although this isn't necessary. Your provider or hospital staff can give you the necessary forms and provide resources explaining the relevant state laws. You can also obtain state-appropriate forms on a variety of websites, such as the National Hospice and Palliative Care Organization.

The forms should come with directions for filling them out. If you have any questions, ask your doctor or an attorney.

You can update your advance directive at any time. In fact, it's probably wise to take a look at your advance directive on a periodic basis, especially if your health status changes.

To change an advance directive, a witness, a notary public or both may be required. Check the requirements in your state. If you move to another state, you may want to update your directive, even though most states will honor directives from other states. Be sure to discuss major changes with those individuals named in the directives and provide them updated copies.

CHAPTER 19

Inspirational stories

Throughout this book we've shared a lot of information. Don't let it overwhelm you. Remember what we said in the beginning: The best way to make healthy changes that will last for a lifetime is to go slow. Choose one aspect of your lifestyle that you would like to improve, and make gradual adjustments until you reach your goal. When you're ready, move on to the next.

It's our belief that if you follow the guidance and advice this book offers, your health will benefit and so will your quality of life, setting you up to fully enjoy your retirement years.

To provide you with some encouragement and inspiration, we share here the stories of a few individuals who are embracing their later years.

MELODEE AND DENNIS

Melodee and Dennis have no interest in acting their ages. One 84 and the other 85, they say they feel much younger.

Melodee says she takes after her grandmother in that she "thinks young." "My grandmother always told me the reason that she was very young for her years is because she didn't hang around with old people!" That may be why Melodee often finds herself spending time with individuals younger than her. She says they help her feel like she's 40 or 50, not in her 80s.

There's no doubt that Melodee has packed many experiences into her lifetime. She got an early start, too, singing professionally at just three years old. Eventually, she performed on Broadway, owned a handful of beauty salons and even served as her town's mayor.

In her late 60s, she entered and won her first-ever state Ms. Senior America pageant. She used her platform to travel around her state talking to seniors about living their lives to the fullest.

"I want to make it to 100," Melodee proclaims. "And my sister does, too. She's two years older than me. And we both said we want to make it to 100 or better. Chances are, we will."

Melodee's and her partner Dennis' love of life shine through as they speak about the people they've gotten to know and the organizations they're involved in. The two spent a decade working with a music exchange program in which they accompanied American students to Finland and hosted Finnish students who visited the United States. They also participate in a program in which they partner with new medical students. The students they mentor become an extension of the family. "One of them married another doctor and they had twins," Melodee says. "They call us their grandparents. It's a thrill."

Melodee and Dennis each have children of their own — Melodee has three and Dennis one. The two were recently at the hospital to welcome Melodee's fifth great-grandchild.

In addition to their volunteer work, the couple enjoys music. They play it in their home all the time, and they frequently attend live musical performances. "It's a pick-me-up to listen to great music," Dennis says. In fact, music is what brought them together. Melodee sings with her son's band. After one of Melodee's performances, Dennis went up to her and said, "When you're finished with your show, I'll buy you ice cream." They've been together ever since.

The two also like to keep their brains sharp by attending trivia nights. At first, they didn't do so well. "They had a lot of questions about the newer music like Taylor Swift and Dua Lipa," Melodee says. "Once we got my grandson involved, we took first place! Sometimes the medical students join us."

For Dennis, a typical day involves work around the house, some volunteer work, and more than a few jokes. Dennis' father might have something to do with his sense of humor. "My father kept a picture of the Greek Grand Dame of the Jersey herd in his wallet," he chuckles. "He kept a picture of his cow!"

Dennis, who grew up on a dairy farm, credits his parents for good genes — they both lived to almost 90. Dennis says he doesn't mind hard work and he likes to keep busy. He spent much of his career setting up and managing credit unions. He says a bout of kidney cancer in 2018 barely slowed him down. He admits, however, that he's stepped back when it comes to snow shoveling. He lets his neighbor, who has a snowblower, deal with much of the snow. Dennis recommends getting to know your neighbors: "Especially the ones with snowblowers!"

The couple's advice to anyone who wants to live younger is to get out, get involved in something, volunteer, and appreciate life. "Our families, our grandchildren, our friends and being a part of a community is wonderful," Melodee says. "And the organizations that we belong to — they give you a reason to wake up in the morning." The two also credit their longevity to home-cooked meals and a lot of laughter.

Melodee sums up their philosophy, "Keep moving. Keep laughing and keep loving."

GEORGE

George doesn't believe that getting older means growing old. He sees too many people who think they need to slow down once they turn 65. He doesn't buy it. "Don't let your mind tell your body you can't do things anymore."

At 74, George likes to keep busy and stay involved. He says it's what gives him purpose. Each morning he takes his medications, practices meditation and does some basic stretching. Then he's off to some type of activity. George attends a chair aerobics class. He volunteers at the local historical society and the local library. He participates in city council activities with a goal of helping to build alliances within the community. He visits his grandson's classroom and reads to the students. He enjoys singing when he can; he's been singing since childhood and once used to sing in a band. Another of George's passions? He likes to talk! He visits with people whenever he can.

For George, healthy aging is all about attitude and outlook. While he doesn't view himself as a religious person, he does consider himself to be a spiritual person. George's life has centered on a few guiding principles, which include keeping an open mind, maintaining an optimistic outlook and, most importantly, practicing compassion and love. He says these basic tenets have served him well through life's ups and downs.

Like many individuals, George's health hasn't been perfect. In fact, he's dealt with several medical conditions during his lifetime, including asthma and heart disease. But George says it was a diagnosis of lung cancer that really forced him to see what he was made of. After a couple of days of feeling sorry for himself, George decided there would be no more moping. He wasn't about to lose hope and let the cancer get the best of him.

George says during his cancer treatment and recovery he thought back to his grandmother, who instilled in his family that giving in wasn't an option. When faced with difficult circumstances she would tell family members they needed to "step up and step out." George, who is now cancer-free, says the experience was another reminder of all he has to be thankful for, and each morning he feels fortunate to enjoy another day.

George credits his family for helping him through difficult times. He's very close to his three adult children and his grandchildren.

George says his health right now is pretty good, and he wants to keep it that way. He lives alone and hopes to for as long as he can. He says even if one day he needs the help of a walker, he doesn't plan to slow down. "That walker will still be moving!" he says.

When people ask George his advice on making the best of their later years, he tells them to keep an open mind and continue to stay active and do what they enjoy. "You've got to live your life."

MARILYN

Marilyn likes to challenge her brain every day — sometimes multiple times a day. The 91-year-old says her love of words and word games keeps her mind feeling young. She's been doing newspaper crossword puzzles for years. "I do that every morning," she says, "except on Sunday. They're too hard." Marilyn also meets a friend every morning for a game of Scrabble. They don't keep score. It's just for fun and good for the brain.

"My mind feels like it's in its 20s. My body is 90, but my legs are 163!" Marilyn quips.

Marilyn says she became fond of Scrabble because it was the only game that she could beat her late husband at. "One time he taught me cribbage, but he'd played it for years, so he was way better than me," Marilyn says, laughing. "He beat me almost every time. I was OK but I'm much better at words."

After her daily Scrabble game, Marilyn takes a walk around the independent living facility where she lives. Despite having bad arthritis, she tries to keep active. For about 20 years, Marilyn met a friend each morning and they walked 3 miles together. "I think that was a really good thing to do," she says. These days she uses a walker and doesn't go as far.

Marilyn says at this stage in her life, keeping mentally fit is easier than keeping physically fit. In addition to her crossword puzzles and Scrabble games, she plays word games online. She also enjoys watching "Wheel of Fortune" and "Jeopardy!" and playing along.

"I don't want to brag, but I'm pretty good at 'Wheel of Fortune,'" she says. "I think it's because I do all those crosswords." She finds "Jeopardy!" tougher. "If I get five in 'Jeopardy!,' I feel like a genius," she says. "'Celebrity Jeopardy!' is a lot easier though. If you want to feel like a genius, watch 'Celebrity Jeopardy!'"

In addition to games, Marilyn keeps her mind sharp by reading. A former pre-school teacher, she loves to read fiction. Her daughter bought her a Kindle reading device, which she uses a lot. "She sees what I buy," Marilyn says, laughing. "And she says, 'Mom, you go from Amish to smut.' In other words, I like everything."

Marilyn credits a positive attitude and good genetics for her health and longevity. She says she tries to look for the positive side of situations and not find fault or make a big deal of inconveniences. For Marilyn, circumstances in life are what you make of them and how you handle them.

"I have only two friends left, so sometimes I say, 'What am I still doing here?' But I'm happy; I am. I think a positive attitude added to this, but an awful lot of it is genes." Marilyn says she's enjoyed good health, and all her medical care throughout her lifetime has been from a general practitioner. "I've never but once been to a specialist," she reflects. "I've really been fortunate."

PAT AND JOE

On New Year's Day in 1951, Pat dared her boyfriend, Joe, to marry her. "We maybe had a little too much to drink," she laughs. Unafraid, Joe accepted. The two of them, along with four friends, piled into one car and eloped to Arkansas. Seventy-two years later, they're still married. Pat, 93, and Joe, 98, raised two children, supporting each other through life's many ups and downs, including the illness and eventual death of their only grandson.

Love and a positive attitude have been keys to their marriage and their health. "You've got to be positive," Pat says. "That's so important in life, and you don't really care about being around negative people. I don't think it's real healthy to be around that too much."

Joe, a former Marine, adds that keeping physically active has helped him age well. "I've played tennis, baseball, football and golf," he says. He also enjoys long walks.

Regular exercise has been a part of Joe and Pat's lives for as long as they can remember. Early in their marriage, Joe and Pat walked to work and around town because they couldn't afford a car. They continued walking because they enjoyed the activity. Joe says he walked 2 miles every day for most of his life — for fitness and to get where he was going. "I'd walk to the golf course, which was up the hill, and back."

Though he's had to adjust his routine in recent years, Joe still prioritizes his fitness. He does some exercises as soon

as he gets out of bed in the morning. Later, he pedals on a stationary bike. In the evenings, he takes laps up and down the hallway of the facility where he and Pat live. Pat reminds him to be careful and focus on his leg strength and balance to avoid falls.

For many years, one of Pat and Joe's joys was visiting their cabin in Colorado. They loved the mountains, wildlife and spending time with friends and family. Only recently, when the high altitude started to affect them, did they stop making their trips to the cabin.

"We've tried to maintain an active life, both mentally and physically," Joe says. When the weather is nice, the two still enjoy being outside. They even keep a garden where they grow tomatoes, green peppers and flowers. "I always plant gerbera daisies," Pat adds. "They're my favorite."

These days the two fill much of their time with hobbies and social activities. Pat is an avid crafter. She knits and paints blown eggs. "I used to decorate maybe 20 a year and give them to friends who had a new baby or new marriage," she says. "I also knit hats for children with cancer. And this fall I knit a large afghan for each of our four granddaughters because they have tall husbands."

A retired lawyer, Joe reads the Wall Street Journal *every day. He says it keeps him mentally sharp. He also enjoys reading financial magazines and articles on his computer. He was an avid reader of books as a younger man but now prefers shorter articles.*

The two also are rabid University of Kansas Jayhawks men's basketball fans. Joe, his daughter and a granddaughter attended the university. "We had season tickets for 10 years and never missed a game," Joe exclaims.

In thinking back on their lives, Pat's take on the secrets to good health are to prioritize what's important to you, dare the man you love to marry you and make room in the garden for the flowers that make you smile.

Additional resources

ADVANCE DIRECTIVES

AGS Health in Aging Foundation

www.healthinaging.org/age-friendly-healthcare-you/care-what-matters-most/advance-directives

American Hospice Foundation

americanhospice.org/caregiving/medical-issues-to-be-considered-in-advance-care-planning/

National Hospice and Palliative Care Organization

www.nhpco.org/

National Resource Center on Psychiatric Advance Directives

nrc-pad.org/faqs/

AGING

AARP

aarp.org

American Geriatrics Society

www.healthinaging.org/

American Society on Aging

www.asaging.org/

National Hispanic Council on Aging

www.nhcoa.org/

National Indian Council on Aging

www.nicoa.org/

National Institute on Aging

www.nia.nih.gov/

ASSISTED LIVING

Administration for Community Living

eldercare.acl.gov/Public/Resources/BROCHURES/docs/Housing_Options_Booklet.pdf

National Consumer Voice for Quality Long-Term Care

theconsumervoice.org/get_help

ELDERCARE

Eldercare Locator

eldercare.acl.gov/Public/index.aspx

EMPLOYMENT

National Experienced Workforce Solutions

www.newsolutions.org

SCORE

www.score.org/

Workamping

www.workamper.com/about/about-workamping

HOUSING

Administration for Community Living

eldercare.acl.gov/Public/Resources/BROCHURES/docs/Housing_Options_Booklet.pdf

American Academy of Family Physicians

familydoctor.org/housing-options-for-seniors/?adfree=true

U.S. Department of Housing and Urban Development

www.hud.gov/topics/housing_choice_voucher_program_section_8

Village to Village Network

www.vtvnetwork.org

INSURANCE

Centers for Medicare and Medicaid Services

www.medicare.gov/Pubs/pdf/10050-Medicare-and-You.pdf

HealthCare.gov

www.healthcare.gov/

Insure.com

www.insure.com/

U.S. Department of Veterans Affairs

www.benefits.va.gov/benefits/offices.asp

U.S. Social Security Administration

www.ssa.gov

RETIREMENT

AARP

aarp.org

Alliance for Retired Americans

www.retiredamericans.org/

Women's Institute for a Secure Retirement

wiserwomen.org/

Index

A

acquired immunity, 128-129
acute inflammation, 129
advance directives, 310-311, 319
aerobic exercise. *See also* exercise
    about, 223
    bicycling, 225
    calories burned by, 228
    types, 225-229
    warming up/cooling down and, 227
age-related changes
    bones, 87-90
    brain, 21-26
    digestive, 101-111
    frailty, 178, 179
    hair, 153-154
    hearing, 50-53
    heart, 61-72
    injury recovery, 179-182
    lungs, 79-82
    muscles and joints, 94-98
    sexual health, 157-159
    sight, 45-48
    skin, 149-150
    sleep, 142-144
    smell, 55-56
    taste, 56-57
    touch, 58-59
    urinary, 117-124
    weight, 136-139
age-related hearing loss, 50
aging
    anorexia of, 112

aging continued

approaches to, 11-12

from birth, 8

cellular breakdown and, 11

cellular clutter and decline and, 13

cellular senescence and, 13-16

chronic inflammation and, 16

disease and, 11

genetic damage and, 12-13

process, 10-16

resources, 320

understanding of, 8

alcohol use

as bladder irritant, 120

bones and bone loss and, 92

cancer risk and, 174

coronary artery disease and, 67

high blood pressure and, 69

immune system and, 133

mental/emotional well-being and, 33

osteoporosis and, 89

stroke risk reduction and, 38

Alzheimer's disease. *See also* brain

changes

about, 24-25

brain changes, 25

plaques and tangles, 25, 26

signs and symptoms, 24

anorexia of aging, 112

anxiety. *See also* depression

exercise as benefit for, 221-222

gut-brain connection and, 107

social companionship and, 200

assisted living, 302, 320

asthma, 82

B

back pain, 96-98

balance exercises, 236-237

behavior assessment, 191-192

behaviors, changing, 192-195

benign prostatic hyperplasia (BPH), 123-124

bladder changes, 118

bladder irritants, 120-121

bladder training, 124-125

blood cholesterol test, 276-280

blood pressure. *See also* high blood

pressure

about, 67-68

classifications, 68

control, 63-64

measurement, 280, 281

sleep and, 78

blood volume, decreased, 64

BMI (body mass index), 137, 138

bone density test, 92-93

bone health, 54

bone loss

about, 87-88

disks in spine, 88

injury recovery and, 181

osteoporosis and, 88-90

bone marrow, 85

bone(s)

age-related changes, 87-88

basics, 83-84

cortical, 85

density, 86-87

fractures, 92, 93

osteoporosis and, 88-90

remodeling, 85
what you can do for, 90-92
bowel movement difficulty, 108-109
brain changes
about, 21
Alzheimer's disease, 24-25
attention, 22
cognitive reserve and, 26
dementia, 23-24
emotional processing, 22
executive function, 22
gut-brain connection and, 107
judgment, 22-23
language, 22
memory, 21
processing speed, 21
responsiveness, 23
that aren't typical, 23-25
brain health
about, 19, 20
brain-friendly foods for, 37
factors in, 27
keys to, 33-38
mental/emotional well-being and, 27-33
neuroplasticity and, 20-21
physical activity and, 34
sleep and, 34-35
social connections and, 35-36
stress management and, 36
tools for offsetting memory changes
and, 38-43
"brain training," 41
breast cancer. *See also* cancer
about, 162
measures influencing risk, 176

risk factors, 163-165
risk reduction therapy, 176
screening, 164
signs of, 162-163
bulging disks, 97-98

C

caffeine, 70, 120
calcium, 89, 90
cancer
about, 161-162
breast cancer, 161-162
colorectal cancer, 168-171
development of, 162-166
diet and, 172-173
lung cancer, 165-166, 176-177
obesity and, 161, 163, 167, 171
physical activity and, 173-174
prostate cancer, 166-168
risk, reducing, 171-177
risky behaviors and, 175
skin cancer, 150-151, 174
tobacco use and, 171-172
weight and, 140
cardiovascular disease
early intervention, 72
progression of, 61
risks, responding to, 74-78
social companionship and, 197
cardiovascular health
about, 74-75
diet and, 76-77
physical activity and, 75-76
sleep and, 78, 145

cardiovascular health *continued*
    smoking cessation and, 75
    stress management and, 78
    weight and, 77-78
care partners, 198-199
cataracts, 46-47
cellular breakdown, 11
cellular clutter and decline, 13
cellular repair, reduced, 130
cellular senescence, 13-16
cholesterol, increase, 62. *See also* blood
        cholesterol test
chronic inflammation, 16, 129, 130
chronic kidney disease, 119-122
chronic obstructive pulmonary disease
        (COPD), 81-82
cognitive health. *See* brain health
cognitive reserve, 26, 35
colon cancer screening, 283-284
colonoscopy, 169
colorectal cancer. *See also* cancer
    about, 168-170
    inherited syndromes and, 170
    risk factors, 170-171
    risk reduction, 177
    screening, 168
    symptoms, 170
conductive hearing loss, 52
congenital heart disease, 70
constipation, chronic, 108-109
coping resources, 212
core stability training, 231-233
coronary artery disease
    about, 64-66
    early intervention, 72
    heart attack warnings and, 65
    risk factors, 66-67
COVID-19, 57, 80-81, 128, 131

D

deafness, sudden, 53
dehydration, 120
dementia. *See also* Alzheimer's disease;
        brain changes
    about, 23-24
    exercise and, 221
    risk factors, 24
    sleep and, 35
dental checkup, 102, 103, 284
depression
    exercise benefits for, 220-221
    hearing loss and, 29
    increase in likelihood of, 32-33
    seeking help for, 33
    symptoms of, 32
diabetes
    colorectal cancer and, 171
    coronary artery disease and, 67
    exercise and, 223
    management, in stroke risk reduction,
      38
    screening, 285-286
    weight and, 139-140
diarrhea, chronic, 109
diet. *See also* Mayo Clinic diet; *specific*
       dietary elements
    about, 249-250
    bone density and, 87
    for brain health, 37

cancer risk and, 172-173

cardiovascular health and, 76-77

colorectal cancer and, 171

coronary artery disease and, 67

gut microbiome and, 106

hearing loss and, 54

immune system and, 132-133

injury recovery and, 181-182

kidney stones and, 123

muscles and joints and, 99

plant-based, 76, 106

prostate cancer and, 167

resilience and, 184

skin and, 152-153

small changes, benefits of, 258-260

unprocessed vs. ultraprocessed foods
and, 259

urinary health and, 125

for your eyes, 49

digestive changes

about, 103-104

bowel movement difficulty, 108-109

fiber and nutrients and, 111-114

GERD, 110-111

gut microbiome and, 104-106

heartburn, occasional, 106

lactose intolerance, 108, 109-110

physical activity and, 115

probiotics and, 114

responding to, 111-116

digital rectal exam (DRE), 287

dry eyes, 45-46

dry mouth, 103

durable power of attorney for health care,
310, 311

E

eating habits assessment, 189-190

electrolyte imbalance, 70

emotional changes, 22, 28

environmental pollutants, 74

estrogen exposure, 89-90, 163

executive function, 22

exercise. *See also* physical activity

about, 215-216

aerobic, 223-229

amount of, 222-223

anxiety reduction and, 221-222

balance, 236-237

benefits of, 218-222, 238

bones and bone loss and, 91-92

cancer risk and, 173-174

core stability training, 231-233

depression reduction, 220-221

disease prevention and, 222

endurance, 219

in firming the body, 218-219

flexibility, 233-236

guide, 237-248

immune system and, 132, 219

importance of, 216-217

increased energy from, 219-220

longevity and, 216, 238

lungs and, 83

mental well-being and, 220

mood and self-esteem and, 222

motivation for, 237-238

physical activity vs., 218

resiliency and, 184-185

skin and, 153

exercise *continued*
    sleep and, 147, 222
    strength training, 91
    stress reduction and, 78, 220
    urinary health and, 125
    water, 225-227
eye exam, 286

F

fall risk assessment, 291
fats, 254-255, 257
fecal occult blood test/fecal immuno-
        chemical test (FOBT/FIT), 283
fiber, dietary, 111-114, 252
financial planning, 297-298
fitness assessment, 190-191
flexibility exercises, 233-236
floaters, 46
fluid consumption, 114, 124
fractures, bone, 92, 93
frailty
    aging and, 178, 179
    resilience and, 182-183
    what you can do for, 183-185

G

gastroesophageal reflux disease (GERD),
        106, 110-111
genetic damage, 12-13
genetics, longevity and, 9, 10
geroscience, 11
glaucoma, 47
goals, in changing behaviors, 194-195

grief and loss, 30-31
growth mindset, 185
gum disease, 102-103
gut microbiome, 104-106
gut-brain connection, 107

H

hair and aging, 149, 153-156
hands-on practices, 266-267
happiness, 185
health span, 14-15
healthy diet. *See* Mayo Clinic diet
healthy weight. *See also* obesity; weight
    about, 136
    BMI and, 138
    portion size and, 115
hearing issues, 51-53
hearing loss. *See also* sensory health
    about, 49-50
    age-related, 50
    conductive, 52
    listening devices, 53
    mental health and, 28-29
    other health conditions and, 51
    sudden, 53
    what you can do for, 53-54
hearing protection, 53-54
hearing test, 289
heart, the. *See also* cardiovascular health
    abnormal response to healing, 63
    about, 60-61
    additional health risks, 72-74
    chronic stress and, 73-74
    function, 61

heart and blood vessel changes
    age-related, 61-64
    arrhythmias, 69
    artery narrowing, 62
    artery stiffening, 62
    blood pressure, 63-64, 67-69
    blood volume, 64
    cholesterol, 62
    coronary artery disease, 64-67
    heart rate, 63
    heart valve disorders, 62, 71-72
    that aren't typical, 64-72
heart attack warnings, 65. *See also*
        coronary artery disease
heartburn, occasional, 106
hepatitis screening, 289-290
herbs and supplements, 268-269
high blood pressure. *See also* blood
        pressure
    about, 67-68
    arrhythmias and, 70
    coronary artery disease and, 67
    exercise and, 223
    injury recovery and, 181
    managing, in stroke risk reduction, 38
    risk factors, 69
    weight and, 140
holistic health
    about, 261
    hands-on practices, 266-267
    herbs and supplements, 268-269
    integration of, 271
    mind-body practices, 262-266
    natural energy practices, 267-271
hormone therapy, 160, 163-164, 176

housing, 299-302, 321
human papillomavirus screening (HPV),
    290
hypercalcemia, 93

I

immune system
    about, 127-128
    acute vs. chronic inflammation and, 129
    age-related changes, 129
    basics, 128-129
    cellular repair and, 130
    conditions that aren't typical, 130-131
    COVID-19 and, 128, 131
    exercise and, 219
    injury recovery and, 181
    sleep and, 134, 144-145
    slower response of, 129-130
    social companionship and, 197
    what you can do for, 131-134
inactivity, 221. *See also* exercise; physical
    activity
independent living, 301
inflammation, 16, 129, 130
injury recovery
    aging and, 179-182
    prehabilitation and, 181
    resilience and, 182-183

J

joint flexibility/function, 95. *See also*
    muscles and joints
judgment, 22-23

K

kidney changes, 118
kidney stones, 122-123

L

learning, lifelong, 43
legumes as fiber source, 255
life span, health span gap and, 14-15
life triggers, 29-30
lifestyle
    healthy, tenets of, 131-132
    longevity and, 9-10
    sedentary, injury recovery and, 180
living will, 310, 311
loneliness, 29
longevity, 8-10, 197, 216, 238
long-term care insurance, 308-310
lung cancer, 165-166, 176-177. *See also*
        cancer
lungs
    about, 79
    age-related changes, 79
    asthma and, 82
    COPD and, 81-82
    COVID-19 and, 80-81
    exercise and, 83
    infection and, 80, 83

M

macular degeneration, 47-48
mammogram, 282-283
massage, 266

Mayo Clinic diet, 250-253
Medicare
    about, 302-303
    coverage, getting, 305-306
    decision-making, 306-307
    original, 305
    Part A, 303
    Part B, 303-305
    Part C (Medicare Advantage), 306
    Part D (prescription drug plans), 306
    private fee-for-service (PFFS) plans,
        306
    resources, 304, 321
medications
    managing, 294-295
    osteoporosis and, 89-90, 92
    polypharmacy and, 295
    sleep and, 143, 148-149
    urinary health and, 126
meditation, 263
Mediterranean diet, 250-253
memory
    age-related changes, 21
    changes, tools for offsetting, 38-43
    sleep and, 144
    tricks, 42
Meniere's disease, 52-53
menopause, 157, 158
mental health, 28-29, 143, 197-200
mental/emotional well-being
    about, 27-29
    depression and, 32-33
    excessive alcohol use and, 33
    hearing loss and, 28-29
    life triggers and, 29-30

social companionship and, 200

stress and, 31-32

mind-body practices, 99, 262-266

mood and self-esteem, 222

muscle mass, 94-95

muscles and joints

about, 93-94

back pain and, 96-98

joint flexibility/function and, 94-95

muscle mass and, 94-95

osteoarthritis and, 95-96

what you can do for, 98-100

N

natural energy practices, 267-271

neurons, 20

neuroplasticity, 20-21

night-shift work, 74

O

obesity. *See also* healthy weight; weight

about, 136

cancer and, 163, 167, 171

coronary artery disease and, 67

high blood pressure and, 69

kidney stones and, 123

obstructive sleep apnea, 70, 140, 293

optimists, 202-203

osteoarthritis, 95-96, 97, 98, 140

osteoporosis. *See also* bone(s)

about, 88

back pain and, 98

risk factors, controllable, 89-90

what you can do for, 90-92

oxidative stress, 12-13

P

Pap test, 286-287

pelvic floor exercises (Kegels), 125-126

peripheral neuropathy, 58-59

physical activity. *See also* exercise

assessment, 190-191

bone density and, 87

brain health and, 34

cancer risk and, 173-174

cardiovascular health and, 75-76

digestive changes and, 115

exercise vs., 218

health and, 217-218

hearing loss and, 54

muscles and joints and, 98-99

peripheral nerve function and, 59

resilience and, 183-184

physical assessments, 189-192

Pilates, 233

plaques and tangles, 25, 26, 35

positive attitude, 185

prayer, 212-213

prehabilitation, 181

probiotics, 114

processed foods, 259

progressive muscle relaxation, 262

prostate cancer. *See also* cancer

about, 166

risk factors, 167-168

screening, 168

signs and symptoms, 167

prostate enlargement, 123-124
prostate-specific antigen (PSA) test, 287-289
provider, working with, 292-294
purpose and health, 205-210

R

reading difficulty, 45
regenerative medicine, 14
religion, 211. *See also* spirituality
resilience
    additional strategies for, 185
    assessment, 192, 193
    daily environment and, 202
    developing, 182-183
    diet and, 184
    frailty and, 182
    health and, 201-202
    optimism and, 202-203
    physical activity and, 183-184
    social connections and, 184-185
resistance training. *See also* exercise
    bands or tubing, 231
    benefits of, 218-219, 220, 229
    bones and bone loss and, 91
    free weights, 229-230
    instruction and safety, 231
    machines and home gyms, 230-231
    plan, 230
    strength and, 231
retinal vessel occlusions, 48
retirement
    creativity and, 210
    finances and, 207

    finding purpose and, 206-210
    hobbies and interests, 208
    key questions, 300
    maintaining identity and, 210
    part-time job in, 209
    planning, 297
    resources, 322
    role models, 207-208
    transition to, 206
    volunteering and, 209
    workamping and, 208
retirement communities, 299-300
rheumatoid arthritis, 97
ruptured disks, 98

S

salivary gland disorders, 57
salt (sodium chloride), 256-258
screening tests
    blood cholesterol test, 276-280
    blood pressure measurement, 280, 281
    bone density measurement, 280-282
    clinical breast exam and mammogram, 282-283
    colon cancer screening, 283-284
    dental checkup, 284
    diabetes screening, 285-286
    eye exam, 286
    frequency, 272
    importance of, 272-273
    optional, 289-291
    Pap test, 286-287
    preventive (men), 279
    preventive (women), 278

PSA test and digital rectal exam, 287-289

recommended, 276-289

self-reflection, 188-189

sensory health

about, 44

hearing, 49-54

sight, 45-49

smell, 54-56

taste, 56-58

touch, 58-59

sexual health

about, 157

age-related changes, 157

conditions that aren't typical, 157-159

dyspareunia and, 160

hormone therapy and, 160

menopause and, 157, 158

misconceptions, 156

risks, responding to, 159-160

shared living, 300-302

sight changes. *See also* sensory health

cataracts and, 46-47

colors and light and, 45

dry eyes and, 45-46

floaters and, 46

glaucoma and, 47

macular degeneration and, 47-48

reading and, 45

retinal vessel occlusions and, 48

that aren't typical, 46-49

what you can do for, 48-49

skin

about, 58

age spots (liver spots), 150

aging and, 149-150

checking regularly, 152

cleansing, 153

examination, 289

health and, 150-153

moisturizing, 153

over-the-counter products and, 154-155

risks, responding to, 151-153

sleep and, 145

sun exposure and, 151-152

wrinkling, 150

skin cancer, 150-151, 174

sleep

about, 141-142

age and, 142-143

bedtime rituals and, 146-147

brain health and, 34-35

cardiovascular health and, 78

exercise and, 147, 222

health and, 144

immune system and, 134, 144-145

importance of, 145-146

injury recovery and, 181

medications and, 148-149

muscles and joints and, 99

naps and, 147

needed, 143

as a priority, 146

worry time and, 148

sleep disorders, 143

SMART goals, 194

smell, 54-56. *See also* sensory health

smoking cessation

bones and bone loss and, 92

smoking cessation *continued*
    cancer risk and, 171-172
    cardiovascular health and, 75
    coronary artery disease and, 67
    GERD and, 111
    high blood pressure and, 69
    immune system and, 133
    lungs and, 83
    osteoporosis and, 89
    sight and, 49
    skin and, 152
    in stroke risk reduction, 37-38
    urinary health and, 126
social connections
    benefits of, 200
    brain health and, 35-36
    care partners and, 198-199
    grief and loss and, 31
    health benefits of, 196-200
    longevity and, 10
    as a priority, 201
    resilience and, 184-185
    spirituality and, 211-212
    support network, building and,
        200-201
spinal stenosis, 98
spirituality
    about, 210, 214
    benefits of, 211-213
    defining, 211
    developing, 213
    health and, 210-213
spouse, loss of, 30
stool DNA test, 283
stories

George, 314-315
Marilyn, 315-316
Melodee and Dennis, 312-314
Pat and Joe, 316-318
Rachel, 6-7
stress and stress management
    brain health and, 36
    cardiovascular health and, 67, 73-74, 78
    exercise and, 220
    gut-brain connection and, 107
    health and, 32
    health risk of, 31-32
    high blood pressure and, 69
    immune system and, 133-134
    longevity and, 10
    muscles and joints and, 99
    strategies, 36, 264
    triggers, 78
stretching, 234-235
stroke risk, reducing, 37-38
**sudden sensorineural hearing loss
      (SSNHL),** 53
sun protection, 48-49, 151-152, 174
support network, building, 200-201

T

tai chi, 237, 270-271
taste, 56-58. *See also* sensory health
teeth and mouth changes, 101-103
thyroid disease, 70
thyroid-stimulating hormone (TSH) test,
    290
tinnitus, 52
touch, 58-59. *See also* sensory health

transferrin saturation test, 290-291
transitions and health, 30, 204-205, 206

U

ultraprocessed foods, 259
unprocessed foods, 259
urinary health
    age-related changes, 177-178
    bladder irritants and, 120-121
    bladder training and, 124-125
    BPH and, 123-124
    chronic kidney disease and, 119-122
    conditions that aren't typical, 118-124
    fluid consumption and, 124
    incontinence and, 119
    kidney stones and, 122-123
    pelvic floor exercises (Kegels) and, 125-126
urinary tract infections (UTIs), 118-119

V

vaccinations, 174-175, 273-276
virtual colonoscopy, 283
vitamin B-12, 59
vitamin D, 89, 90-91
volunteering, 209

W

weight. *See also* healthy weight
    age and, 136-139
    assessment, 189
    BMI and, 140-141

    health and, 139-140
    heart attack and, 140
    risks, responding to, 140-141
    sleep and, 145
weight loss, 140-141
wellness vision, 187-188
workamping, 208

Y

yoga, 235-236, 262-263

| Mayo Clinic Press

Health information you can trust

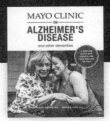

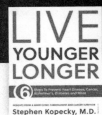

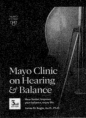

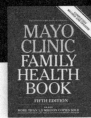

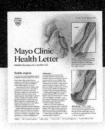

Mayo Clinic on Alzheimer's Disease and Other Dementias

Live Younger Longer

Mayo Clinic on Hearing and Balance, Third Edition

Mayo Clinic Family Health Book, Fifth Edition

Mayo Clinic Health Letter

At Mayo Clinic Press, we believe that knowledge should be shared, especially when it comes to health and medicine. Through printed books and articles, ebooks, audiobooks, podcasts, videos, and more, we provide reliable health information designed to empower individuals to take an active role in their health and well-being.

Our health publications are authored by teams of medical experts, including physicians, nurses, researchers and scientists, and written in language that's easy to understand.

Here is just a sample of some of our other titles:

- Arthritis
- Back and Neck Health
- Mayo Clinic Diet

- Digestive Health
- Prostate Health
- Home Remedies

- Osteoporosis
- Cook Smart, Eat Well
- And many more

Scan to learn more

Discover our full line of publications: **MCPress.MayoClinic.org**